Contents

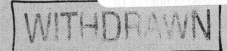

Free companion material

Readers can access additional companion material for free online.

To access companion material please visit:
www.bpp.com/freehealthresources.

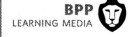

About the publisher

BPP Learning Media is dedicated to supporting aspiring professionals with top quality learning material. BPP Learning Media's commitment to success is shown by our record of quality, innovation and market leadership in paper-based and e-learning materials. BPP Learning Media's study materials are written by professionally-qualified specialists who know from personal experience the importance of top quality materials for success.

About the editors

Dr Aimee Aubeeluck, CPsychol

Aimee is a Registered Practitioner Health Psychologist who has been working in Nurse Education since 2005 at the University of Nottingham. Her research interests include quality of life for patients and their caregivers, communication and global learning initiatives.

Susan Thompson

Susan qualified as a Registered General Nurse in 1986 and has been working in healthcare ever since. She has experience in medical and surgical nursing, critical care, health promotion and nursing management. She has worked both in acute hospitals and community services. She has a master's degree in Public Health and is currently working as a lecturer in Adult Nursing at the University of Nottingham.

Gemma Stacey

Gemma is a Lecturer in Mental Health at the University of Nottingham. She qualified as a mental health nurse in 2004 and has maintained her practice in a community mental health setting giving her current applied knowledge and experience of mental health nursing practice. Gemma's PhD research explores the experiences of Graduate Entry Nursing students in practice.

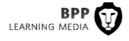

About the contributors

Paula Dawson is a Lecturer in Child Nursing at the University of Nottingham.

David Charnock is a Lecturer in Learning Disability Nursing and Health Promotion at the University of Nottingham.

Justine Barksby is a Lecturer in Learning Disability Nursing at the University of Nottingham.

Anne Felton is a Lecturer in Mental Health Nursing at the University of Nottingham.

Gail Mitchel is an Associate Professor in Adult Nursing at the University of Nottingham.

Emma Taylor is a Staff Nurse who graduated from the University of Nottingham in 2011.

Nicola Siddall is a Staff Nurse who graduated from the University of Nottingham in 2011.

Zoe Smith is a Staff Nurse who graduated from the University of Nottingham in 2011.

Alison Barnard is a Financial Support Supervisor at the University of Nottingham.

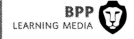

Foreword

As most nurses will tell you, you never really know that you want to be a nurse until you do it. However, you would be silly not to find out as much as you possibly could before taking the first step into your new career. After five decades in nursing I have never regretted taking that one small step to make a giant leap to become a Registered Nurse. The authors of this book have similar and great experience and are abundantly qualified and proficient to offer the sound advice you need. They make clear that as a nurse you will be challenged by the demands of providing nursing care in a compassionate manner but you will also care about being a nurse. Nursing will put you in a privileged position of providing the short- or long-term care for an individual who is unable or lacks the ability to care for themselves.

If you have the motivation, energy and fundamental attributes to become a nurse then this book will lay in front of you the diverse fields of nursing open to you. You could choose to nurse the younger person (child field) or the expanse of the young to very elderly adult (adult field). You may wish to care for those who find it difficult to understand and learn new things and struggle to cope in society (learning disability field). Finally, you could focus on those in mental distress (mental health field). Preparing for registration as a nurse in the UK involves aspects of all these fields with an emphasis on just one of your choice.

The book makes clear that you will need to acquire specific knowledge, skills and attitudes. This will be demanding and challenging, and will also be necessary throughout your career as life-long learning is a fundamental requirement of all professions. The blend of academic and practice pressures you encounter as a student nurse, while being continually assessed, are explored and how this moulds you into a fully-fledged Registered Nurse. You will be left in no doubt about what to expect. Practical and essential information is provided so that you can survive and thrive in the stimulating world of a student nurse.

Finally, I would like to wish those of you who choose to pursue nursing as a career the undoubted privilege of meeting wonderful people during a time of need and the pleasure of working with fantastic and dedicated colleagues.

Peter Davis MBE

MA, CertEd, Bed, RN, DN, ONC
Associate Professor of Nursing – University of Nottingham
Emeritus Editor – *International Journal of Orthopaedic*
& Trauma Nursing

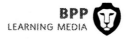

Shining a light on your future career path

The process of researching and identifying a career that you are most suited to can be a somewhat daunting process, but the rewards of following a career that truly engages you should not be underestimated. Deciding on your future career path should be viewed as a fun and extremely satisfying process that, if done correctly, will benefit you greatly.

Carefully considering a short list of future career options and what each one will offer you will help you to make a truly informed decision. Although it is perfectly acceptable to change career direction at a later date, reviewing the options open to you now will help to ensure that you are satisfied with your career from the outset.

I first began mentoring aspiring professionals eight years ago when it was clear that many individuals were not gaining access to the careers guidance they required. It was with this in mind that I embarked on publishing our *Becoming a* series of books, to provide help, support and clear insight into career choices. I hope that this book will help you to make an informed decision as to what career you are most suited to, your strengths and your aspirations.

I would like to take this opportunity to wish you the very best of luck with identifying your future career and hope that you pass on some of the gems of wisdom that you acquire along the way, to those who follow in your footsteps.

Matt Green

Series Editor – *Becoming a* series
Director of Professional Development
BPP University College of Professional Studies

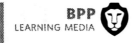

Introduction

Aimee Aubeeluck, Susan Thompson and Gemma Stacey

There are many reasons why you might be considering a career in nursing, for example, because you care about others and want to make a positive impact to individual lives and contribute to society. You may be driven to do something with your life that improves others' quality of life and reduces pain and suffering. You may feel it is your 'calling'. In addition, you may believe you have the key skills that nurses require, such as the ability to communicate and build relationships, empathy and understanding and lots of dedication. Nursing is an exciting and challenging career for men and women of all ages. Starting a nursing career will open many different doors for you and provide you with a variety of opportunities whatever your area of interest or chosen field of study. There are very few careers that offer so many different pathways, such a wide range of different areas to work in and the chance to make a real difference to the lives of others. Key principles of all nursing practice, in whichever field, is respect for patients, a commitment to maintaining their dignity, an ability to empathise with them and be compassionate.

As you decide whether nursing is the career for you, you will have to consider whether your own thoughts and ideas about what nursing is and what nurses do reflect the reality of nursing practice. Nursing is a well known profession, after all many children play 'dress-up' as nurses when they are little. Because nursing is so much in the public eye, there are general perceptions in society of the work nurses do and the type of people they are. Nurses also suffer from stereotypes – administering angel, battleaxe or more salacious images are commonly reported in the media. This book aims to distance itself from these and provide you with a true picture of nursing, thereby enabling you to make an informed choice as to whether nursing is the career for you.

You will have to decide which field of nursing practice you would like to train and work in once registered. This book provides a comprehensive overview of the role of the nurse in healthcare today. It gives the reader insight into nursing as a multi-dimensional profession which reflects the needs and values of society and endeavours to meet the health requirements of individuals and communities. It demonstrates, through nursing theories, practical examples and personal stories, how the

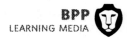

role of the registered nurse is dynamic within the changing context of healthcare provision, requiring a caring approach to professional practice and commitment to working within a multi-dimensional health care environment. It provides the reader with a clear, up-to-date and practical guide to the fields of adult, mental health, child and learning disability nursing linked to the latest Nursing and Midwifery Council (NMC) standards. Readers will gain an insight into the journey of becoming a nurse, from the admissions process into nursing, the student nurse experience and lastly into the role of the nurse in modern healthcare today.

How to use this book

The individual chapters in this book will help you to make several important decisions including:

- Which field of nursing
- Which type of programme
- Which university
- What personal adaptations are required to be successful

Student stories appear in each chapter to give you a first-hand account of what life is like as a student nurse.

The stage you are at in considering nursing as a career will influence how you use this book. If you are in the early contemplation stage each chapter will be informative and insightful. By reading the book as a whole you will gain a clear picture of the options available to you. However, you may be at a stage where you are already clear upon certain aspects and therefore specific chapters would be of use. The diagram below will help you to identify what stage you are at.

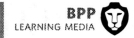

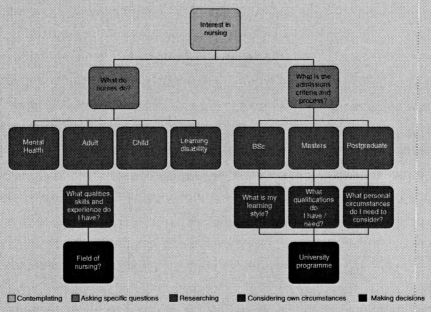

Contemplating ▢ | Asking specific questions ▨ | Researching ▨ | Considering own circumstances ▨ | Making decisions ■

Figure A: Identifying the stage of your journey

Chapter summaries

Chapter 1 Insight into the field of adult nursing

This chapter aims to describe the role of the adult nurse and the client group that adult nurses care for. It discusses the skills adult nurses need to acquire and provides you with an insight into a typical day in the life of an adult nurse. It also gives you an idea of the diversification of roles associated with adult nursing and career pathways you may be able to pursue with an adult nursing qualification.

Chapter 2 Insight into the field of mental health nursing

This chapter will aim to introduce the role of the mental health nurse, identify the nature and focus of mental health nursing and enable you to consider if mental health nursing is for you. The key principles and skills revolve around enthusiasm and commitment to communicate effectively and work collaboratively with people who are often vulnerable and experiencing emotional distress. Job satisfaction comes from comforting a person, supporting them towards their recovery or maintaining their safety in the least restrictive environment possible. It requires the nurse to work with uncertainty, distress and disappointment at times however the opportunity to truly make a difference to an individual and their family happens in every encounter.

Chapter 3 Insight into the field of child nursing

This chapter will identify the nature and focus of child nursing and enable you to consider whether child nursing might be the right career choice for you. As a child nurse you need to be able to assess each child's stage of development in order to tailor your care appropriately. Child nursing involves working in close partnership with parents, carers, a range of professionals and the child themselves.

Chapter 4 Insight into learning disability nursing

This chapter aims to discuss learning disabilities and explore the role of the learning disability nurse. It discusses different aspects of learning disability nursing and the concept of holistic care. It provides real-life stories from both learning disability student nurses and registered learning disability nurses to provide an insight into the day-to-day care work of the learning disability nurse.

Chapter 5 Learning for practice and learning in practice

This chapter will aim to introduce the learning theories which underpin nurse education programmes and describe the different types of approaches adopted when learning in the university and practice settings. The ways in which teaching and learning are interpreted and implemented will vary across the different universities, so it is important to identify the structure and format of the courses that you are considering. We hope that the information here will help you to ask the right questions to ensure you reach a decision which best fits with your personal learning style and requirements.

Chapter 6 Choosing the right course for you and making a successful application to university

This chapter aims to provide you with the specific information you require to identify the right university course for your needs. It will highlight the stages of the recruitment and selection process and provide you with some tips that may increase your chances of putting together a successful application.

Chapter 7 Mature or graduate entry nursing

This chapter specifically addresses the needs of the mature learner, those over the age of 21 and / or with an existing degree. It will discuss both the benefits and challenges of being a mature entrant,

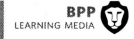

and suggest ways that mature entrants can plan for the changes that embarking on a nurse education course will bring, especially with regard to juggling family commitments and finances. The chapter also discusses graduate entry nursing, programmes for those candidates with existing degrees who may be able to use their existing practice and educational experience and skills to undertake a two-year pre-registration programme.

Chapter 8 How do I manage my finances as a student?

This chapter will give an overview of how to manage your finances as a student, drawing on the personal experiences of student nurses who give top tips on how to survive.

Conclusion

This helps you plan for the commencement of a pre-registration nurse education programme – the course which will provide you with the qualification of registered nurse within your chosen field. It contains an action plan to allow you to fill the gaps in your knowledge and move forward into nurse education.

Chapter maps

The chapter maps below will help you to identify which chapters are relevant to the specific questions you are asking.

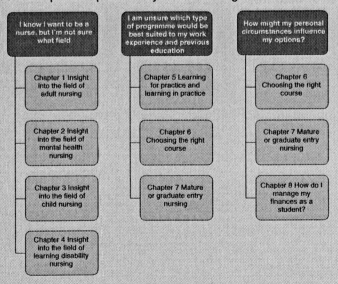

Figure B: Chapter maps

Chapter 1

Insight into the field of adult nursing

Sue Thompson

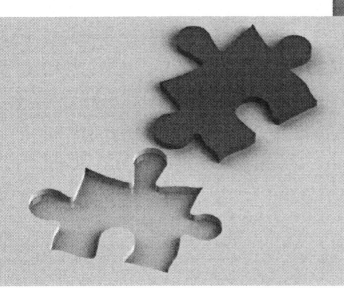

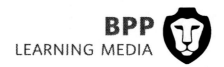

BPP
LEARNING MEDIA

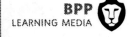

Introduction

Nurses working in the adult field care for adults generally from the age of 18 years upwards, although most of their client group will be in the older age range. As an adult field nurse you will find yourself working with patients from all levels of society and from all ethnic groups, all with differing health beliefs and values. Adult field nurses care for patients with very differing needs and conditions in a variety of settings either in the hospital or in the community. You may work on a surgical unit, caring for someone undergoing a brief surgical procedure, a hernia repair for example. From this intervention the patient is likely to recover completely and have no further problems. Alternatively you may be working on a medical ward, caring for people with chronic long-term conditions such as a lung condition which causes breathlessness for example. Many such patients will need continuing care which may involve hospitalisation during periods when their condition worsens for a time. Once stabilised these patients are discharged home to be cared for by community nursing teams who monitor and manage the patient's care to ensure that maximum quality of life is achieved. You may work with adults who have a sudden illness, following a stroke for instance, working alongside occupational and physiotherapists to aid the patient's rehabilitation and helping them to regain their independence. You will need to perfect excellent assessment skills to quickly judge a patient's condition and have the confidence and skill to respond appropriately especially in an emergency situation. An important part of your role will be to care for dying patients and their relatives, ensuring that your patient is comfortable and pain free. In all these roles, in common with other nurses, adult field nurses work to a strict code of conduct (Nursing and Midwifery Council, 2009), having a duty of care to their patients, and relatives and respecting and co-operating with their colleagues.

Assess your skills: What makes a good adult field nurse?

As you'll have a key role in co-ordinating care for patients and will liaise with healthcare professionals from different disciplines, as well as creating a comfortable and caring environment for your patients and their relatives, you will need excellent communication skills. You will need to be flexible and be able to adapt to changing circumstances quickly. Ability to prioritise, good assessment skills and staying calm under pressure are all essential skills, as well as possessing a high level of motivation to ensure that you deliver the best level of care possible. All nurses need to care in the traditional sense of the word and to be able to truly empathise with patients and relatives. Good nurses possess all the above and more, making them highly skilled professionals, but they are also approachable, not hiding behind their status, but willing share their knowledge and work alongside patients and relatives as equal partners in care. The intrinsic skills mentioned above are just as important as the ability to carry out procedures and have knowledge of diseases, treatment and medication for example.

If the above looks daunting don't let it put you off, let's face it, you may already possess these skills to a greater or lesser degree. Self awareness and reflection play a big part in nursing and perhaps it's good to start here, before application. After all a common questions at interview is, 'So why do you want to be a nurse?' or 'Why do you think nursing is the profession for you?'. Successful candidates are more likely to be those who have considered the demands of the role carefully and matched it to their own personal qualities and abilities as well as their interests.

What types of role may my qualification in adult nursing lead to?

All nurses assess, plan, implement and evaluate evidence-based care but this can happen in a wide variety of practice settings. Of all the fields of nursing, the adult field is perhaps the most diverse. Once you have completed a period of study and gained first level registration as a registered nurse, the opportunities are endless. As UK registration is recognised by other European Union (EU) countries, adult field nurses are eligible to work throughout the EU and are usually able to work further afield. The nursing profession is committed to ongoing professional development, so throughout your career, you have the opportunity to work in many different areas of practice and will be helped to extend your qualifications within these specialities.

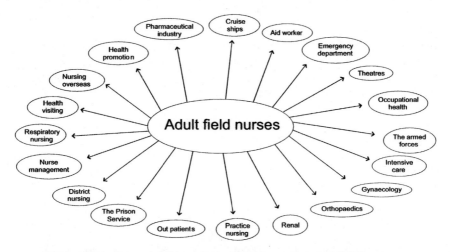

Figure 1.1: Some of the many roles open to adult field nurses

What practice placements should I expect to experience when I am training to be an adult field nurse?

The Nursing and Midwifery Council (NMC) stipulates that all student nurses spend 2,300 hours in practice in order to gain enough skills and experience to allow them to practise as registered nurses. The NMC and the European Union (NMC, 2004) have stipulated that all adult nurses should have had the following practice experiences during their training:

- General and specialist medicine
- General and specialist surgery
- Care of children
- Maternity care
- Mental health and psychiatry
- Care of older people
- Home nursing

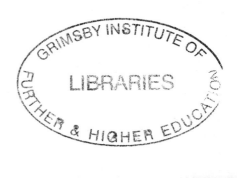

So your programme should contain these areas. However there is no stipulation on the amount of time you should spend in these areas and exactly which practice areas students experience will vary and depend on local circumstances. As a general rule, the bulk of your placements will be on medical, surgical and older people units, with perhaps six to eight weeks on a district nursing placement and between one-and four-week insight experiences on the other areas, but it varies between universities and local health service providers. Large regional centres will be able to provide more specialist placements than smaller centres, however having too much specialism early on can be a handicap, depriving you of seeing the norm, rather than the unusual. Your centre may also provide a learning disability placement which can provide a very useful insight into the health needs of a significant proportion of the population and one which you are sure to encounter during your career. We suggest that you enquire about the practice placements you are likely to experience when you attend for interview.

'I was so excited to get out on to the wards and start practising some of the skills I had learnt in university. It was quite nerve wracking at first but after I had gained the experience, I looked for any opportunity possible to get involved. It gives you quite an adrenaline rush being able to do more hands on skills and provide nursing care to your patients.'

Top tip

In adult field nursing your main client group will be older people so make sure you both like and can relate to older people before you apply.

Try to get work or volunteering experience in healthcare before applying. This will enable to gain a taste of the healthcare environment and judge whether it is right for you. Many hospitals and nursing homes will have vacancies for healthcare assistants. Nursing agencies operate nursing banks employing healthcare assistants on an ad hoc basis therefore providing you with experience and insight rather than a full-time position. Also remember voluntary organisations such as the Red Cross and the St John Ambulance service who are always looking to train volunteers.

Case study: A typical day in practice for an adult field nurse

The title of this section is a misnomer as no day in nursing is ever like another, which is what makes the profession so interesting, yet also challenging. However, days do have structure to them, but this depends on where you will be working. Below is an example:

If you are working on a general hospital ward, the day usually begins with a handover from the shift presently on duty – in the morning this will be from the night shift. Its aim is to ensure continuity of care, a seamless transition of care from one care giver to another, safeguarding the patient's safety and making sure any changes in the patient's condition or care planning have been documented and reported to the nurse who will be taking over the care of that particular patient. This happens in various ways and written as well as verbal communication is necessary so aspects are not omitted or forgotten.

The next thing is to introduce yourself to the patients that you are looking after and work out a plan of care with them for the day. This will obviously vary, perhaps the patient is to undergo a surgical procedure or test for which they will need preparing, or maybe it is planned that they will go home that day, or perhaps they are still quite poorly and require regular observation and monitoring of their condition. If a new patient is admitted to the ward or unit, you will need to complete a health needs assessment from which a plan of care for that particular patient will be developed.

On a general ward, nurses help patients with their hygiene needs, their nutrition, their mobility, their toileting needs and many other things. Roper, Logan and Tierney (2000) describe such needs as '*Activities of Living*'. Other typical duties include the issuing of medication, urinary catheter care, maintenance of intravenous fluids, bed-making, meeting with other healthcare professionals involved with the care of your patient, removing surgical drains, taking blood pressure, temperature, pulse and respirations – the list goes on.

During care giving, nurses continually reassess their patient to ensure that the plan of care for that patient is still appropriate and as a consequence the plan will be amended accordingly. A key factor in this is liaison with other health professionals involved in the patient's care such as doctors, physiotherapists, dieticians, social workers etc. Much of a nurse's role is connected with helping patients to acquire the skills that they need to care for themselves, skills that they will need once they go home. You may for instance teach a patient and their relative stoma care and how to empty and renew a colostomy bag, ensuring the patient's skin remains intact and doesn't become sore.

Documentation of care given and changes to that care is an essential legal requirement for nurses. While there are plans for such documents to be computerised in the near future, many care plans are still on paper. Therefore readable handwriting and clear and concise expression are key requirements for nurses. The shift ends as it began, with you handing over the care of your patients to the nurse who has been assigned to them for the next shift. You will need to be concise, give specific details as necessary and be 100% accurate.

Learning adult field nursing in universities

During your time at university, you will be taught the principles of adult field nursing. As you may have gathered, care of adult patients is a vast area of practice. Nurses therefore are generally are taught within a symptom rather than a disease framework, care of the breathless patient for example. Of course nurses are given knowledge of common medical conditions and their treatment, but it the nursing care of the patient that is the focus. Care needs to be holistic, ie treating the patient as a whole individual and therefore encompassing all aspects of the patient's life that their condition will impact upon. This may be their mobility and nutrition, but also perhaps their social and sex life.

Care also needs to be evidence-based, ie proven through research to be effective, and student nurses are taught in school how to access reliable evidence and also how to critique research to ensure that it is of a high quality and is unbiased. Unlike doctors, nurses generally do not diagnose, although nurses initiate and amend nursing care and more senior and specialist nurses can hold their own caseload, prescribe medication within a defined formulary of drugs, as well as performing a range of clinical procedures.

Nurse education programmes need to demonstrate robust links between teaching theoretical concepts of care and the transfer of this into actual nursing practice on placement areas. The use of real-life scenarios and simulation can help bridge the gap that sometimes can occur between theory and practice. Good links between the university and practice areas with nursing lecturers both visiting and working on placement areas also facilitate students' learning and ensures taught sessions demonstrate current practice.

All student nurses are assigned a mentor during their time on a placement area. Mentors are registered nurses who help you to identify learning opportunities in practice and oversee and assess your clinical progress and competence. Student nurses are taught essential clinical

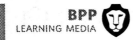

skills such as how to safely handle and move patients, how to take basic observations of temperature, pulse and respiration, how to ensure infection is not transmitted from patient to patient, how to administer medication to patients etc. Such clinical skills are taught in school and practised in placement areas. However as well as adopting a caring role it is stressed that patients are partners in care: an important aspect of the nurse's role therefore is to impart knowledge and skills to patients and their relatives. Patients are also assisted to adopt lifestyle changes and nurses act as health promoters and educators. Skills such as assessing and increasing a patient's motivation to change and supporting them in the process are important aspects of the role.

Generally nursing programmes are made up of modules or sections, each with a particular emphasis which reflects the student's level of training and experience. Basic nursing care and key nursing principles may for example be the focus of the first module, whereas management and leadership is most likely to be the focus of the last module. Assessment varies between university programmes but range from assignment or essay writing, to written exams, group or individual presentations and short clinical examinations in which specific skills are assessed.

Programmes again vary as to how much of the programme is shared with other fields of nursing, such as mental health and children's nursing and how much is just with your adult field counterparts. There are pros and cons to this. All adult nurses will need to nurse adults with mental health problems or adults with learning disabilities when they develop a physical health problem. People do not fall neatly into boxes, so it is important for adult field students to have a basic understanding of the needs of all groups in society. However it is also important the shared learning does not 'water down' the clinical skills you as an adult field nurse will need to possess at a higher level than a mental health nurse for example. Therefore it is useful for the programme to offer specific field sessions as well as shared field sessions.

Chapter summary

Adult field nursing is a rewarding and interesting profession. Of all the nursing fields it is the one that allows for the most scope for different practice experiences including working in other countries. Because of its tremendous variety it can appear daunting as there is so much to learn. However during your nurse education you will be taught key principles and skills which are transferable to all areas of practice.

Key points

- On qualification adult field nurses have the opportunity to pursue a wide variety of roles.

- Adult field nursing is challenging, both physically and mentally. Adult field nurses juggle the needs of their patients with the need to organise and manage their ward or community area.

- Adult field nurses need skills in assessment and care, communication and liaison, administration and research as well as being clinically competent and able to respond sensitively to the needs of their patients and their carers.

Useful resources

The role of the adult nurse:

www.nhscareers.nhs.uk
www.rcn.org.uk
www.nmc-uk.org

Castledine, G and Close, A (2009) *The Oxford Handbook of Adult Nursing.* Oxford: Oxford University Press.

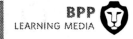

References

Nursing and Midwifery Council (2004) *Standards of Proficiency for Pre-registration Nursing Education.* London: NMC.

Nursing and Midwifery Council (2009) *Code of Conduct for Nurses and Midwives.* London: NMC.

Roper, N, Logan, W and Tierney, AJ (2000). *The Roper-Logan-Tierney Model of Nursing: Based on Activities of Living.* Edinburgh: Elsevier Health Sciences.

Chapter 2

Insight into the field of mental health nursing

Gemma Stacey

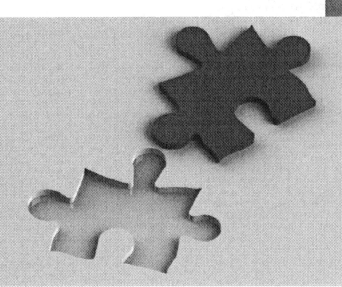

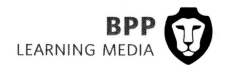

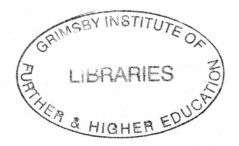

Introduction

This chapter introduces the role of the mental health nurse, identifies the nature and focus of mental health nursing and will enable you to consider if mental health nursing is for you.

Mental health nursing is an extremely varied and wide-reaching profession. Mental distress is acknowledged as a major health issue in the 21st century and is therefore a high priority for every healthcare worker. As a nurse in a mental healthcare setting you would have the opportunity to work alongside people who are experiencing mental health problems and accessing mental health services. For some people their distress impacts on their quality of life to such an extent that they require additional support. This is often provided by mental health nurses working as part of a team of other professionals such as doctors, occupational therapists and social workers. For some people the combination of the experience of mental distress, using mental health services and society's perception of mental health problems has excluded them from participating in the roles and activities in society that most people would take for granted.

The work of the mental health nurse is stimulating, challenging and dynamic. It requires an appreciation of the impact of social inequalities and injustice to understand a person's distress within their social context. This understanding informs mental health nursing practice and requires the nurse to respond on a psychological, physical and emotional level. The way this might be achieved is not prescriptive and may be influenced by a number of different theories, clinical skills, and organisational philosophies. It is also dependant on the individual relationships that are fostered between the nurse and the person requiring support. The nature of these relationships will be influenced by both your own and the person's beliefs, values and attitudes. Commitment to developing an awareness of these and effective interpersonal skills are, therefore, at the core of mental health nursing.

What is a mental health nurse?

Mental health nurses work across many diverse settings including GP's surgeries, Accident and Emergency departments, community teams and in-patient psychiatric wards. However, there are core skills and values which are integral to this work whatever the setting. Mental health nurses are involved in working directly with individuals and families to provide support and deal with the impact of being diagnosed with a mental health problem. They are involved in promoting the health of the individual but also increasingly working with schools, colleges and communities to promote mental health and enable people to access opportunities outside mental health services to maximise their potential. Mental health nurses are also involved in managing and leading care and contributing to the improvement of healthcare through research and the development and implementation of strategies for enhancing quality.

You may have come across debates surrounding the focus and boundaries of the mental health nursing role. This has been influenced by the origin of mental health services, the rapidly changing context of healthcare over the past 50 years as well as the lack of agreement as to the exact cause and therefore best treatment of mental ill health. This culminates in a situation where it is perhaps more difficult to answer that important question 'what does a mental health nurse do?' than it initially seems.

This is reflected in the following descriptions of a typical day for a mental health nursing working in an in-patient and community. These examples are fictitious however they do reflect the usual routines of these environments.

Case study 1: Typical day on a mental health older adults ward

Safire Ward (older adults ward for people with memory problems)

6.50   Arrive for early shift

7.00   Receive a handover from the night shift

7.45   Support the healthcare assistants with helping the patients get washed, dressed and serving breakfast

9.00   Administer morning medication and complete physical observations for people who require them

10.00 Discussion with the doctor regarding a number of patients who require medical review

10.30 Make a phone call to a social worker who is currently assessing the financial circumstances of a patient on your ward to gain feedback on its progress

10.45 Spend time in the communal area of the lounge having informal chats with the patients and gaining an impression of their general wellbeing

11.30 Meeting with a patient's husband who has concerns about how he will care for his wife when she is discharged home. He becomes tearful and you spend some time comforting him and explaining to him the support that will be provided.

12.00 Support the healthcare assistants with serving lunch and observe how one of the patients is managing to eat. You then document this in the patient's ongoing nutritional assessment.

1.00 Administer lunch time medication

2.00 Spend one-to-one time with a new patient who has recently been admitted and is expressing a high level of anxiety. You begin to engage with her and to build a formulation of her precipitating factors and consequent thoughts which occur when feeling anxious.

3.00 Write up the clinical activity of the shift in the patients' notes taking into consideration any changes, assessment made or liaison with other services while your colleague hands over to the staff on the late shift who have just arrived.

Case study 2: Typical day in a community mental health team

Diamond community mental health team

9.00 Arrive at the office to collect the medication you will need to administer that morning. This is stored in a locked case which you put in the boot of your car.

Log the visits you are planning for the day in the dairy to enable the team to check your whereabouts and safety.

9.45 Head out to visit James Wilson who has a long history of using mental health services and a diagnosis of schizophrenia. You are preparing for him to be discharged from the service and working with him on a relapse prevention plan.

10.30 You drive to visit Christine Jones who is a new referral and requires an initial health and social care assessment. You are visiting her at home with a colleague who is a social worker to begin the assessment process.

12.00 You return to the office to give feedback on the assessment and several others you have recently completed to your team in a referral meeting. You jointly decide the care package for Christine and begin to write a letter to her GP to inform them of the plan of action.

2.30 You go to the local GP's surgery to meet one of your clients who has diabetes and is not managing it well. You provide her with support to discuss her problems with the GP and agree on a management plan which you will jointly implement with the practice nurse.

3.00 You stay at the GP's surgery to run a medication clinic where a number of service users come to have their medication administered by injection and discuss their general wellbeing.

4.30 You return to the office to document the clinical activity of the day in the patient's notes.

As you can see from these examples the setting in which you work as a mental health nurse will highly influence the nature of the day-to-day work. However, there are fundamental elements of the role which will now be discussed.

What does a mental health nurse do?

Top tip

The best way to answer this question is to speak to people who are mental health nurses or who have had contact with them. You could also look at the following websites which would give you an indication of the types of issues you are likely to be dealing with as a mental health nurse.

- Bob the Psychiatric Nurse
  ds.dial.pipex.com/bob.dunning/bobthe.htm
- MIND
  www.mind.org.uk
- Rethink
  www.rethink.org

The therapeutic relationship

The main tool that the mental health nurse has at their disposal to impact positively on an individual's health is his or her self. The relationship that a nurse and person who may experience mental health problems establish is, therefore, central. This means that

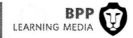

communicating effectively and learning to really listen and understand another is one of the most important aspects of being a mental health nurse. Without this the support a nurse is able to provide is limited. Through the therapeutic relationship mental health nurses assess, plan, implement and evaluate care. This is structured through individual time spent with the person.

Assessment

Using interpersonal interaction and sometimes using more formal assessment tools the mental health nurse will be involved in a process of assessment with the individual experiencing mental distress. This will entail developing an understanding of what it is like to be that person at that point in their life. Integral to this is gaining a holistic perspective which will incorporate an exploration of their mental distress and current problems but also the impact of relationships, social situation, culture, physical health, spirituality and their strengths and coping strategies on their current experiences and future hopes and goals.

Planning care

The nurse will then work with the individual and potentially their family to prioritise the support that they require and develop a plan of care outlining the nature of that support. What this will entail and the resources that it will incorporate will clearly depend on the individual, their experiences and the context in which care is being delivered.

Interventions

Outlined below are the areas where a mental health nurse may provide support, followed by some examples of what this might mean. This is commonly known as areas of intervention.

Practical	Accessing benefit entitlements or supporting someone with an application for a educational course
Social	Gaining information and helping people to access community resources (such as groups, clubs, courses, gym) and social opportunities to reduce isolation, extend social networks and enhance self esteem. It may mean going with them to these activities
Psychological	Exploring the different ways that the individual may cope, helping them to identify what might trigger or make their distress worse and consider different ways of coping that they may not have tried before
Biological	Administering medication alongside outlining support for an individual to regularly monitor their blood sugars for diabetes or plan for supporting an individual who may self-harm by dressing their wounds
Spiritual	Enabling people to access the resources and opportunities that create meaning in their life. This may entail providing a safe space for the person to explore the meaning of their experiences of mental distress

Table 2.1: Areas of intervention

The mental health nurse will be engaged in this continual process of assessment, planning, supporting or providing an intervention, evaluating the impact of this and re-assessing to inform the next process. This is developed in collaboration with the individual and, where they are involved and consent is given, family and friends. The involvement of the person experiencing mental health problems within this process is essential to ensure that the care provided is meaningful and relevant to them. There are times when this collaboration is challenging such as when care is enforced through the individual being detained under the mental health act or when a person is so distressed that direct communication about care is difficult. This is a potential tension within mental health services and the role of the mental health nurse.

Is mental health nursing for you?

The following will help you to consider if this field of nursing is of interest to you. The statements below identify the key attributes of a mental health nurse and the level to which you agree with them will give you some indication of your suitability for the role.

Assess your skills

- Building relationships with people is my main motivation for considering nursing as a career.
- I believe in the potential of people to change and grow.
- I feel passionate about advocating for people who lack a voice in society.
- I feel confident in my communication skills.
- I am able to listen to people's problems without expressing judgement.
- I am able to consider a situation from a range of perspectives.
- I am able to empathise with a person's situation even if I do not agree with their behaviour.
- I am comfortable engaging with people who express unusual thoughts or bizarre beliefs.
- I am comfortable engaging with people who express extreme sadness or lack any motivation.
- I am aware that I may be involved in enforcing treatment against a person's will if they are assessed as lacking the capacity required to make an informed judgement.
- I am committed to learning about myself and how my personal values may influence my practice.

The following accounts given by mental health students exemplify their motivation and passion for selecting this area of practice.

As you read these accounts consider if you would feel equally dedicated and enthusiastic about the type of clinical work they describe.

'Mental health field allows me to talk to people about their past history and how they can move forward to create a different future. It allows me to hopefully make a difference for them and their families, which is so rewarding. Before arriving at my first mental health placement I remember being genuinely scared about what to expect. I worried that maybe mental health nursing was not for me and maybe I had made the wrong decision. However, within five minutes of being there I remember realising that mental health is definitely the right decision for me. I found it fascinating watching the people in their day-to-day lives and finding ways to help them and move forward. It was an enriching experience to have, and has changed the way I think about things in so many ways.' **Amanda Smilie**

'There are always lessons to be learned and trials to go through. The real reward is going through someone else's trial with them, being allowed in under the wall that they put up for everyone else. Somehow because you suddenly are called a nurse they believe that you care and as long as you don't convince them otherwise they will let you care for them. That may be holding their hand when they're distressed or listening when they feel so isolated but when someone does let me in it confirms that I'm in the right place, I've found my 'calling' as it were.' **Fredrick Lee**

'The encounters that I have had with patients experiencing dementia, schizophrenia and depression have all been as unique as the individuals themselves and have offered both challenge and delight. Validation that I had finally chosen the 'right' path came when, during my first placement, an elderly lady gripped my hand for comfort after she had taken a stumble, and equally so, when an acutely depressed young man with whom I had worked in the community, told me, with all the excitement of a teenager experiencing their first flush of love, about his new relationship.' **Helen Moran**

'The most challenging experience for me so far has been trying to engage a service user, with a diagnosis of personality disorder, in activities to try to distract her from self harming. This was a very long task, which at times I wanted to give up on. However, I persevered and in the end it became my most enjoyable moment as the service user engaged well with the activity and did not self harm that day.'
Kathryn Greenwood-Lambert

Career prospects

As a mental health nurse your career can take you in many directions. These can vary from providing direct care in a ward or community environment, developing skills in specific therapies to become a specialist nurse practitioner or leading services through management roles. The client group you could be working with can also vary significantly from children and young people with behavioural problems, adults with criminal convictions who also have mental health problems or older adults with memory problems to name just a few. The stories below are written by mental health nurses who have experience of working in the varied areas of practice.

Case study: Ruth Pretty – Child and Adolescent Mental Health Services (CAMHS)

'I have worked as a mental health nurse in CAMHS for the past ten years. The main part of my work is giving therapeutic support to children and young people when they are experiencing mental health difficulties. I can work with the young person alone or with them and their family. I also include other agencies involved in the young person's life such as teachers, social workers or workers from voluntary agencies. The work is very varied and every day is different. For example next week my diary includes appointments with a young mum at home who is too scared to take her baby out for fear of germs and illness; a girl who has restricted her food intake so much that she is now dangerously underweight; a six-year old recently diagnosed with autism who is feeling very angry, and a young man who is feeling suicidal after experiencing two bereavements.

The thing people most often tell me when I say what I do is that they couldn't do it because they would find it too upsetting to work with children who have had bad experiences. At times it can be distressing to enter the lives of those who have experienced abuse, loss or trauma but I find the worst part is usually reading the reports of some children's histories. When you meet the child or young person you feel amazed at how resilient they are; you see their strengths and you find hope. Some of the challenges of the job are trying to get everyone to work together to help the young person (it tends not to work when this doesn't happen) and having to accept that sometimes it is just not the right time for the young person to get support. The rewards are the privilege of being part of a young person's and their family's life during such a sensitive and precious time, and feeling that you have contributed to a young person's recovery. I think it helps to be open minded, compassionate, playful, genuine, able to get on with people from all walks of life and to have a good sense of humour.'

Case study: Rosie Robinson – Staff Nurse, rehabilitation in the voluntary sector

'I have been qualified for around 18 months and am working for a charity called Rethink Mental Illness. They provide a number of services for people who struggle with mental health difficulties, this can be from housing projects to support lines. I work in a rehabilitation unit which strives to maintain people's daily living skills and support them to set goals they wish to achieve. The people that I work with have severe and enduring mental health needs and have been identified as needing 24-hour nursing support. My role as a nurse working for Rethink Mental Illness on a day-to-day basis involves a lot of organisation and management of time and staff. I can often be the only nurse on the unit and therefore have the responsibility of being in charge of the safety of those using the service and those working in it. I have a group of four service users with whom I work using the recovery model to identify how they currently feel in all areas of their life and what they wish to change. I then support them to do this by structured goal planning.

One aspect of my job which may differ from other nursing roles is that Rethink has a strong campaigning arm which attempts to challenge the stigma of mental health. This has involved me going out to the local area with information about mental illness and getting people talking about mental health. I also liaise with other professionals in the community, for example the police who are due to come to give a talk to our service users on the effects of racism in the community.

I think my most important role as a nurse is that of an advocate for those that use the service. My lead area is involvement, meaning that I am continually looking at ways to involve our residents in the decisions made about the care they receive. When a new member of staff is being hired for Rethink we give our residents the opportunity to be part of the interviewing panel and formulate questions beforehand focusing on what is important to them. I also conduct a residents' meeting every month and make sure that the residents' views and wishes are taken into consideration when shaping the service.

I think that my role is so much more than you expect when you hear the word "nurse", but this is both challenging and rewarding. Supporting people to be independent and involved in their care every step of the way gives me a satisfaction that I could not achieve in any other profession.'

Case study: Susanna Morris – Community Mental Health Nurse

'I went straight into working as a community mental health nurse after finishing my degree four years ago, and I have stayed as it really suits me and I enjoy it so much. It is a privilege to be invited into people's homes and get to know them.

As a Community Mental Health Nurse / care co-ordinator, my role is very varied, and although I work as part of a team, I get to bring in my own individuality and style of working. No week looks the same and my diary rarely goes to plan due to the unpredictability of my patients' circumstances and team issues. I work with people aged 18–65 with severe and enduring mental health issues. This can include bipolar disorder, chronic depression, schizophrenia, personality disorders, anxiety, post traumatic stress disorder, and eating disorders. I liaise with psychiatrists, psychologists, GPs, social workers, hospitals, schools, housing officers, benefits departments, voluntary agencies, support staff, OTs, the police, other mental health departments, and out of area units. This is to make sure everyone is working together who needs to be involved in supporting my patients. I have the responsibility of regularly performing risk assessments and formulating care plans and often need to act as an advocate for my patients to other agencies and professionals. I also have other responsibilities such as ordering medication, developing the recovery focus of our team, giving injections, organising support for carers and mentoring students. I have also trained in Behavioural Family

Therapy which I use to support families to improve their communication skills.

I thoroughly enjoy working with so many different individuals and their families, using kindness and compassion, as well as clear thinking, assertiveness and academic knowledge. It feels so worthwhile to help people achieve and live a full life despite their mental health needs and I enjoy the creativity needed to plan care around an individual's needs, lifestyle, and preferences.

While the job is exciting and rewarding, it can also be very challenging. This can be because of the current financial cutbacks, and other issues which come hand-in-hand when working for a large organisation like the NHS. I regularly have to talk to people about issues like self harm and suicide, and unfortunately I have had first-hand experience of the effects of suicide, but I try to channel these bad experiences into making sure I value individuals, put them first in their care and provide a quality service. We have a great team spirit and are there to support each other through the challenges.'

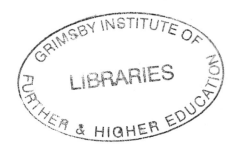

BPP
LEARNING MEDIA

Chapter summary

The insights given in this chapter provide you will some indication of the role of the mental health nurse and the varied focus of this field of nursing. The key principles and skills revolve around enthusiasm and commitment to communicate effectively and work collaboratively people who are often vulnerable and experiencing emotional distress. Job satisfaction comes from comforting a person, supporting them towards their recovery or maintaining their safety in the least restrictive environment possible. It requires the nurse to work with uncertainty, distress and disappointment at times however the opportunity to truly make a difference to an individual and their family happens in every encounter.

Key points

- The role of the mental health nurse is extremely varied depending on the environment and client group you are working with.

- The therapeutic relationship represents the core feature of mental health nursing and a commitment to engaging with people in distress is an essential attribute.

- Communication represents the key clinical skill in mental health nursing.

Useful resources

Barker, P (2008) *Psychiatric and Mental Health Nursing: The Craft of Caring.* 2nd edition. London: Arnold.

Bonham, P (2004) *Communicating as a Mental Health Care*r. Cheltenham: Nelson Thornes.

Callaghan, P, Playle, J and Cooper, L, eds. (2009) *Mental Health Nursing Skills.* Oxford: Oxford University Press.

Clarke, V and Walsh, A (2009) *Fundamentals of Mental Health Nursing.* Oxford: Oxford University Press.

Norman, I and Ryrie I (2009) *The Art and Science of Mental Health Nursing: a Textbook of Principles and Practice.* 2nd edition. Maidenhead: Open University Press.

Chapter 3

Insight into the field of child nursing

Paula Dawson

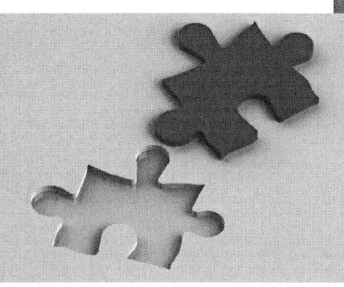

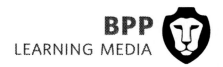

Introduction

Child nursing is a varied, challenging and very rewarding career choice. This field of nursing encompasses a wide age range of clients: those from just a few hours old to those on the threshold of adulthood with 16 or 17 years of life experience behind them.

As a child nurse you will be involved with initiatives to support an individual's health and wellbeing in their own home, at school, within a range of community settings and also within the many areas of a hospital.

Some health needs of those who will be cared for by child nurses will be similar to those of clients within other nursing fields. General, complex and more critical medical and surgical needs can develop across the entire life span, as can mental health problems and those associated with learning disabilities.

Many health problems, some of which will be life-long or life-limiting, will first appear during infancy, childhood or adolescence, and the child nurse has an important role in supporting a child and their family to find the best possible way through the implications and potential effects of their own particular health journey. Neonates, infants, children and adolescents also encounter many conditions which are at the 'cutting edge' of new development and care possibilities. Diagnosis and treatments for some conditions which, one or two generations ago, were certain to lead to death in infancy or childhood have now developed to the extent that many of those with these conditions are reaching adulthood.

The child nurse will work in close partnership with parents, carers, a range of professionals and the child themselves throughout the care experience to promote understanding, involvement and ultimately confidence so that the child and family can make their own decisions about their health needs.

This chapter will:

- Introduce the role of the nurse for children and young people

- Identify the nature and focus of child nursing

- Enable you to consider whether child nursing is the right career for you

What is child nursing all about?

Perhaps the two most significant elements of child nursing which mark it out as a specific and discrete nursing discipline are the following:

- You are caring for individuals who are in a state of continuous change and development.

- As you care for these individuals you are also working alongside, and in very close partnership with, the child's parent(s) and / or guardian(s).

Bearing these elements in mind at all times is essential for the effective nurse. Let's consider what this really means for the practitioner.

The developing child

The child nurse needs to have an in-depth knowledge and understanding of developmental theory and be able to apply this knowledge effectively in their nursing practice. Developmental theory provides a range of frameworks against which the practitioner can determine optimum communication and care plans, individualised to the specific needs of any individual child and family. For example, when considering how and when to explain to a four-year-old what will happen when they go to the operating theatre the nurse will need to consider that a four-year-old is likely to be in the concrete-operational stage of cognitive development, as identified by Piaget (Mitchell and Ziegler, 2007), and will be unable to grasp the abstract concept of something in the future which will be a completely new experience. Attempting to communicate similar information to a 13-year-old will need very different tactics! The child nurse will need to use their knowledge base, their ingenuity and imagination, and their sensitivity to each individual child's temperament and fears, to determine how best to approach each encounter.

The nurse and family working in partnership

When nursing the infant, child and young person it is probably best to acknowledge that you are also going to be 'nursing' their family unit. National policy (Department of Health, 2004) and child health literature (Smith and Coleman, 2010), acknowledge that children should, wherever and whenever possible, receive care at home, surrounded by their own family unit, in the company of their parent(s) or main carer(s).

Most child health areas operate with a policy of open visiting, encouraging parental presence whenever possible and as wished for by the child and family. Obviously, this philosophy has to take account of the child's own individual rights to privacy and dignity, and their developing capacity to determine for themselves exactly who they would like to be where and when.

As a child nurse you will need to get used to working alongside parents and families every step of the way. This can be very daunting, but is also one of the most rewarding elements of child nursing. Providing skilled, confident and highly competent nursing care to sick children, being

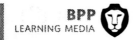

someone in whom they and their parents can place their trust, can learn from, confide in and build their own confidence in collaboration with, is something that can provide great job satisfaction.

What does a child nurse actually do?

As a child nurse, in whichever area of care you undertake your work you will:

- Build a professional relationship with the child and their family.

- Assess the child's health needs in discussion with the child themselves (if they are able), their parent(s) or guardian(s), and other health professionals, such as physicians, surgeons, physiotherapists, occupational therapists, health visitors, school nurses, general practitioners, specialist nurses, play specialists.

- In consultation and negotiation with the child, family and other professionals, plan an appropriate care programme to optimise the child's health and wellbeing, taking account of their age, developmental level and all elements of their usual and expected activities of living.

- Work closely with the child, family and other professionals to action this programme of care, demonstrating evidence-based, highly skilled and competent care methods to do this.

- Record and report all nursing activity using appropriate theoretical frameworks and communication skills.

- Review, evaluate and plan further care activity as and when required in each situation.

- Hand over care management of child and family to other professionals and or discharge the child to the care of their family when your responsibilities have been fulfilled and disengage from child and family appropriately.

Is child nursing for you?

Comments on child nursing, from those who are there...

The comments below are selected to show a range of themes and opinions from practising child nurses, educators and child nursing students currently in employment or studying.

Why did I decide to become a child nurse?

'I have always enjoyed working with children. When I got to a point in life where I was considering a change of career I wanted something practical that made a difference and to work with children. Nursing seemed to offer what I was looking for.'

'There are many reasons why I decided to become a child nurse but more than anything I knew I loved being around children, coming from a very family orientated background just encouraged me to pursue a career in this area. I could not envisage doing anything else.'

'Without sounding at all "cheesy"'I have always wanted to make my mark in the world and to give something back to other people in some way. I have always had a caring nature, enjoy meeting new people and I am extremely ambitious. Child nursing allows me to achieve all of this and more.'

'I found it was just what I loved doing – caring for children and their families in a friendly environment where the staff worked really well together.'

'I had previous work experience within a hospital and found the children's wards had a more positive outlook on treatment and recovery. Children seemed to deal better with illness and recovery.'

'I worked in a nursery with children and trained as a nursery nurse – and I also completed time as a volunteer in a learning disability hospital for children and grew to realise that child nursing would be the right direction for my career.'

The best things about child nursing for me are:

'The children, and knowing that I am making a difference even as a student whether practically or by being able to be supportive to someone who is distressed or upset.'

'Working to help and support children and young people is the best thing about this type of nursing, so for me they are the best part of the job. But because I love being around children and young people so much, for me it does not feel like a job. One day they will be the adults of today's future society, so I feel privileged to be able to work with this group of people and use my role as a future nurse to support and empower them.'

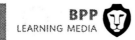

'Everyone works closely with the health and wellbeing of the child in mind. It is very rewarding to see children get better. It is also very rewarding to be able to relieve the stresses of having a sick child for their family and carers.'

'Being able to contribute to the development of the health of children and their parents and interacting with children that have a great deal of enthusiasm for life.'

'Knowing that a good recovery means a better life for the child as they grow older. Knowing they have a lot of life ahead of them to enjoy if their health is good.'

'As a child nurse in practice – the contact with children and their families.'

'As a ward manager of an adolescent unit – the contact with young people.'

'In my career as a child nurse educator – working with people of all ages who wish to become child nurses in supporting the professional standards I know are so important for child nursing, and working strategically with expert child nurses who can lead child nursing nationally and internationally.'

What I enjoyed most about my initial nurse education:

'Well, haven't finished my initial training yet but meeting other people with a similar passion and being able to take what I learn in theory and apply it to help someone.'

'Personally I enjoy meeting new people and talking to them, it is not always possible to have the time as a staff nurse to do this, so I really loved opportunities to play with the children, talk to them about any worries and answer any questions. Also to talk to the families and gain valuable insight into their life as a family, it really helped to develop a professional bond and a sense of trust.'

'I have also had some fantastic mentors who have truly inspired me and developed my confidence so much. They believed in me from the start and supported me through my placement to achieve everything I have to date.'

'The variety of places in which you can nurse children. It was good to see the variety of wards, and community placements as well as being able to go into a range of homes – and realise that even in deprived areas parents love their children just the same as those in wealthy areas... they may just need a different kind of help from nurses to keep their children healthy.'

'The variety of wards that I worked in gave me a great insight into a lot of children and their associated problems. Being able, at a very early stage, to interact with children and their parents and perform skills that were useful at the time. Being able to do simple things with children, such as reading a book or playing a game, helping them to be less scared of being in hospital.'

'The opportunities to learn clinical skills and to understand different areas of nursing for children. Building relationships with children and their families, who were often a long way from their homes.'

What are the essential qualities a child nurse needs to have / develop?

'Patience, a sense of humour, being non-judgmental and having an understanding of people and the fact that not everyone sees things as you do or will feel the same way. You need to be able to make allowances for people's background, experience, abilities, etc, while at the same time putting the child's needs first.'

'Strong communication skills are one of the most essential qualities you will need to have and continue to develop. Take time to talk to your patients and engage with their families in particular, they know their child better than anyone else and you are responsible for the most precious thing in their world, so make them feel included in their child's care. You should also be a good listener, the patient and their family / carer are your focus and you should not be reflecting on your opinions or experiences. Your life experience should be seen as a positive thing, it allows you to show empathy to your patients and their families and to structure the care and support to meet their needs.'

'Skills such as good organisation, time keeping, strong enthusiasm and willingness to learn are essential. No one person will ever hold all of the qualities needed prior to starting their nursing training, there is so much to learn and areas you will need to continue developing throughout your nursing career.'

'To keep the child at the centre of their care. To be an advocate for the child and family. To develop a professional style of working while maintaining an emotional link to those you are caring for.'

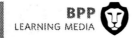

'A sense of humour helps.'

'Patience, understanding, sense of humour and an ability to talk to a child on their level. Being honest with the child and parent and a great imagination to be able to find alternative ways of caring, when met with a child who is afraid of procedures.'

'A good knowledge base – really understanding the physiological, psychological, sociological (including ethics and law) and pharmacological knowledge for child nursing – and how to apply the knowledge base in different situations.'

'Calmness and empathy and the capacity to ask if unsure, recognising one's own limitations.'

'Excellent communications skills.'

The most difficult element of child nursing for me is:

'Sometimes seeing parents who just don't seem to care or understand what their child needs.'

'The most difficult part of child nursing is that you will come across situations that may be upsetting and challenging, where you may feel enough is not being achieved by either the family or professionals. I found this very difficult at the beginning of my nursing course and I have been involved in circumstances that were upsetting at times. The most challenging aspect of this is biting your tongue, but this does comes easier in time. You need to be open-minded and unprejudiced no matter how difficult, and provide every patient with the same degree of compassion and equality in care.'

'Sending children back into environments that I know they will not thrive in.'

'Seeing a child that will not recover well enough to enjoy the remainder of their lives. This is comparative to children of the same age. Helping children and their parents come to terms with long-term health issues.'

'Supporting parents in coping with diagnosis, and managing child death. Always different, mostly challenging...'

What makes child nursing different from other nursing fields?

'The focus on family – most children are part of some form of family unit and you have to treat them as part of that unit. It is not just about looking after the child or considering their needs, though you have to be an advocate for them, but considering them as part of a family and caring for the family.'

'The main difference in child nursing from other types of nursing is you are not just thinking about a patient but also their wider family, carers and friends. You have to consider the impact your decisions will have on the family unit and work in partnership to achieve the care plan goals.'

'It is a more relaxed style of working, with less of a hierarchy within the working team. The range of patients is the widest you could possibly have, and as a result you develop a very wide range of skills. It is also very demanding – especially when caring for very sick or dying children.'

'There is a sense of happiness as most children will recover fully. Also there is a greater involvement with the child and family to influence future development. Almost like being able to help them prevent any problems in the future through health education input.'

'You are working with those for whom life and understanding is developing and changing very rapidly in many ways, and your stance in caring must reflect this.'

If I could describe the experience of child nursing to someone who is considering it for their own career, what would I say?

'It's hard work and at times heartbreaking, you go home wondering what is going on in some families and what's going to happen to a child, but it's also so worthwhile and you meet so many lovely families.'

'I have realised that the biggest difference you can make is often just by accepting people, having a kind word or a smile or a cup of tea! Listening to their worries and doing what you can to relieve them. And sending home a well child is amazing!'

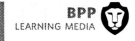

'When I am having a tough day the moment that always sticks in my head is when a young patient who I had looked after very closely came up to me on discharge, with a picture she had drawn for me and kissed my hand to say thank you for looking after her. Her parents also gave me the biggest thank you and told me I would make a fantastic nurse. This meant the world to me and I still have that picture today.'

'These are the moments that make all the challenging days feel insignificant and remind you of why you chose to be a child nurse. I am now in my second year; I am still nervous and have a lot to learn but feel I am starting to get somewhere in my education and will one day make a real difference.'

'It is enjoyable working with children that have a zest for life, and illness does not always have to be a bad time. Being able to help in the development of a young life and assist in the recovery and return to good health to enjoy for a long time.'

'Child nursing is tough – practically and emotionally difficult at times – but rewarding and you have the real chance to contribute to changing lives. You need to be well prepared and you need to realise that it is not always about giving care, but having the ability to have the knowledge and the sensitivity to support families to be able to provide best care for their children. This can be challenging as a student, but it is worth the challenge.'

'I would say that it is a great career choice and I am thrilled to have been chosen for the position. The work load isn't easy but the outcome is worth it.'

Top tip

Child nursing is a hugely rewarding career in which you will meet many amazing children, families and colleagues. However, working with sick, distressed and vulnerable infants, children, young people and their families can also be very challenging, making this a career choice that needs careful consideration.

Assess your skills: Have you got what it takes?

Consider whether you feel that you have these qualities and skills:

- A compassionate and caring nature
- Great communication skills with people of all ages and from all walks of life
- The ability to work as a team member and also independently
- The ability to listen and take the trouble to consider how you may help people in the way that will suit them best
- Good organisational skills
- The ability to use your own common sense and initiative
- A determination to constantly develop your professional knowledge and skills

These important qualities and skills are by no means an exhaustive list of those you will need as a child nurse, but if you choose to follow this path you will need to demonstrate these attributes on a daily basis!

Case study: My life as a child nurse

'My experience of child nursing has provided some of the most challenging experiences of my life but they are also some of the most rewarding moments. If you enjoy meeting new people, have a caring nature, enjoy being around children, thrive on a challenge, want experience working in varied settings and learning new skills every day from different professionals, then child nursing could be for you. It is a career choice which is never dull or boring. Every day, every encounter will be different. I have been fortunate to work in many places around the UK and also in Europe and Africa, in roles which have required me to develop a huge range of skills; from delivering excellent 'hands-on' nursing care to children, and leading and managing a staff team, to offering teaching and support to children, parents, staff and colleagues.'

Chapter summary

This chapter has introduced you to the role of the nurse for children and young people and provided some information about the nature and variety of work which a child nurse may undertake. It clearly highlights that one of the most striking features of child nursing is how often you share your skills with others. Your job is to give the child's carers the confidence and ability to carry on with the caring role at home; it's all about knowing when to stand back and when to take over if necessary. Child nursing is tougher and broader than some imagine it to be, but there is plenty of evidence that those who choose this career path find it enormously rewarding.

Key points

As a child nurse you will:

- Care for individuals from infancy to adulthood, dealing with a very wide range of health issues

- Work in very close partnership with the child and the child's parent(s) and / or guardian(s)

- Encounter sad and stressful situations, such as children with life-limiting conditions, children who have been harmed, and children who die

- Encounter many examples of courage, bravery and humour

- Work very hard, in a very supportive environment, as part of a motivated professional team

Useful resources

Bird, J and Borrego, M (2010). *Nursing and Midwifery Uncovered*. 3rd edition. Surrey: Trotman Publishing.

Hall, C and Ritchie, D (2011) *What is Nursing? Exploring Theory and Practice*. Exeter: Learning Matters.

www.nhscareers.nhs.uk

www.nurses.co.uk

References

Department of Health (2004) *Children's National Service Framework for Children, Young People and Maternity Services.* London: The Stationery Office.

Mitchell, P and Ziegler, F (2007) *Fundamentals of Development: the Psychology of Childhood.* Hove: Psychology Press.

Smith, L and Coleman, V (2010) *Child and Family-Centred Healthcare: Concept, Theory and Practice.* 2nd revised edition. Basingstoke: Palgrave Macmillan.

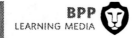

Chapter 4

Insight into learning disability nursing

Justine Barksby and David Charnock

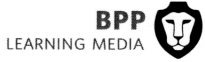

BPP
LEARNING MEDIA

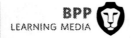

Introduction

The role of the learning disability nurse is a unique and challenging one. It is an area of nursing that is truly multifaceted, interesting and varied. As discussed later in this chapter the nurse is required to use a holistic approach to care, which addresses every aspect of a person's life. Learning disability nursing is a small area and perhaps one of the least known and least understood, which possibly reflects the status of our client group. Many people do not understand what learning disability means and so before we discuss the role of the learning disability nurse, we need to explore what we mean by 'learning disability'.

Definition: Learning disability

One definition of learning disability is:

- 'A significantly reduced ability to understand new or complex information, to learn new skills (impaired intelligence), with,

- A reduced ability to cope independently (impaired social functioning);

- Which started before adulthood, with a lasting effect on development.'

(Department of Health 2001, p.14)

It is important to remember that people with learning disabilities can learn, but they sometimes have difficulty when something is new to them or if it's just too complicated. Nurses may help to reduce the complexity or help the person to interpret the world around them. Also, people with learning disabilities may have problems in social situations or when they have to deal with other people. It may be that the nurse needs to help the person to learn how to communicate more effectively with other people or to understand their condition, an aspect of which may make it difficult to understand the approaches of others. Finally it's important to note that learning disability nurses work with people of all ages, but the learning disability must have been diagnosed before they reached adulthood.

Sometimes people with learning disabilities have conditions such as Down's syndrome or autistic spectrum disorder, which requires the nurse to work in special ways to assist the person and their family or carer. Some people with learning disability live independently with minimal support while others need 24-hour care. Often people with learning disabilities have other conditions or diseases including physical disabilities or mental health problems which impact directly on how they are affected by their learning disability, how they are viewed by others and how complex their care might be. The individuality of learning disability, its presentation and ability range, make the role of the learning disability nurse extremely diverse.

This chapter will:

* Explore 'learning disabilities' and learning disability nursing

* Look at the role of the learning disability nurse

* Help you decide if you have what it takes to be a learning disability nurse

What is a learning disability nurse?

Background / history

The role of the learning disability nurse has changed significantly over the last 25 to 30 years, as too have the lives of people with learning disabilities. In the past people with learning disabilities faced a life removed from mainstream society, along with others identified as unsuitable, blamed for many of the problems that society faced. As people with learning disabilities were often seen as unable to provide for themselves, the image cast was that of people who were a burden on the state (Wright, 1996). This has led to the misconception that in the past the majority of people with learning disabilities were abandoned by their families and institutionalised. This is not the case and as Walmsley and Rolph (2001) have argued, the lives of people with learning disabilities have largely been a part of family life and community care; institutional care should only be viewed as part of a continuum of care and not as the sole model. However, the care of people with learning disabilities whether in institutions, the home or the community was governed by a strict regime of care and control that restricted all aspects of their lives (Walmsley and Rolph, 2001). People with learning disabilities were not free to do as they or their family wished, as they were required to register and comply with a rigid set of rules.

The 1960s heralded a change in the way people with learning disabilities were cared for. Driven by a number of scandals in large institutions and a growth in social theory, the restricted lives of people with learning disabilities was seen as preventing them from living as members of society. Consequently, there has been a great deal of scrutiny over the years regarding the lives of people with learning disabilities and the role of the nurses who support them. Despite the questions asked about the role of specialist nurses for people with learning disabilities over the last four decades, the specialism has survived. People with learning disabilities now live in the community and the service provided by learning disability nurses is community based.

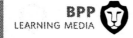

'My motivation to begin working with people with learning disabilities was the belief that I could help someone change their lives. It's a small world and I like the fact that I still see people I worked with when I started my first staff nurse post. It's good to catch up about what's happened to us over the years.'

Holistic care

Holistic care means addressing every aspect of a person's life. In some areas of nursing the nurse is concerned with a small aspect of the person, such as the illness or condition; in learning disabilities the nurse works to support and develop the whole person.

Learning disability nurses are, of course, concerned with their physical health and this is a huge part of their role but equally they address mental / psychological / emotional needs; they care for a person's social wellbeing and address spiritual or sexual needs.

Sometimes people with learning disability may make unwise decisions and they may lack the capacity to understand the consequences of these decisions due to their learning disability. As a nurse you may support a person in this situation. Consider the following example: a person you are working with decides to wear his favourite shorts, the only problem is, it's January. What are the risks associated with this decision? Think in terms of the physical risks but also the social implications. What would you do?

What does a learning disability nurse do?

'This year I celebrated my 20th year in learning disability nursing and I can honestly say I have never regretted a day! There have been some challenging days, a few stressful days but many, many great days.'

As mentioned previously, the role of the learning disability nurse is a diverse one and consequently the role is conducted in a range of service settings. Within NHS provision this can range from community-based teams to secure hospital services. Across the range of provision, services can include Assessment and Treatment teams, health facilitation teams and health access teams. Learning disability nurses also work in private and charitable organisations which broaden the role further still. This diversity makes the role a difficult one to define however some definitions include: liaison with the multi-disciplinary team and co-ordinating services, communication skills, management skills, and direct care. On one hand learning disability nursing can involve broad diverse responsibilities, but on the other specialist / focused roles in epilepsy, challenging behaviour, forensic services and continence advice (Manthorpe *et al*, 2004). These components highlight some of the differences in the role: often in private services the role will be a broad care provider role whereas in the NHS services the role is more of a specialist focusing on a specific healthcare need or condition.

Learning disability nursing is different to many areas of nursing as it does not work within a 'sickness' model of nursing (Mitchell, 2004) because in many areas learning disability nurses are enabling and empowering people who are physically well.

Further elements of the role have been described as:

- Health and promotion of autonomy (Kay *et al*, 1995)
- Agents of inclusion (Gates, 2002)
- Autonomy and health promotion (Moulster and Turnbull, 2004)
- Health facilitator (Valuing People, 2001)

(all cited in Mitchell, 2004).

It also involves:

- Teaching new skills
- Family support
- Team working
- Enabling clients to access services
- Co-ordinating services to meet client needs
- Finding 'places' to suit skills and aspirations

(Bottomer, 2004)

Northway *et al* (2006) when talking about the future of the role stated:

> *'Learning disability nurses will lead the way in achieving positive health outcomes for people with learning disabilities. They will use an inclusive and collaborative approach to address barriers to social inclusion and will function as integral members of the wider family of nursing, developing and using specialist knowledge and skills to improve health and wellbeing of children, adults and older people with learning disabilities across all settings.'*

Although there are many similarities, these defining elements show the multifaceted nature of what it is to be a learning disability nurse, demonstrating its uniqueness as a profession. Learning disability nurses are adaptable, helping to build services around the individual; not changing the person to fit the service. Having a learning disability means that you experience difficulty integrating into society – the nurse's role aims to create the pathways to enable that to happen and put the person at the centre of their lives.

Some people with learning disabilities communicate through alternative methods such as signing or symbols and nurses need to be able to engage in these methods of communicating too. Imagine you are hungry or thirsty but are not able to get food or a drink yourself. What would you do? Most of us would ask. Imagine then, if you could not communicate in a way that those around you understood. How do you think you would feel? What would you do? This simple example illustrates the importance of having a system of communicating that those around us understand.

In recent years reports have highlighted the health inequalities people with learning disabilities experience when accessing mainstream health services, including abusive practices and poor care where the very basics of care were omitted, such as food and drink (Mencap, 2007; Michael, 2008). These tragedies have led to the creation of roles for learning disability nurses as health facilitators, supporting people with learning disabilities to access mainstream health services and supporting the staff of these services in order to ensure equitable care for all.

Assess your skills – Is learning disability nursing for you?

- Can you think on your feet?
- Can you be spontaneous?
- Can you juggle the complexities of risk and vulnerability with advocating and empowering people?
- Can you communicate in alternative ways?
- Can you be a role model for others?
- Can you initiate change and challenge systems?

This chapter has described the role of the learning disability nurse – not a simple task due to the wide range of roles they fulfil – but it should have given you an understanding of what learning disability nursing can involve. To illustrate this further below are some accounts from learning disability student nurses about why they chose learning disability nursing:

Case study: Diane Sheppard (third year student): 'My journey to becoming a learning disability nurse has not been a simple one. When I first started college six years ago I had ideas of becoming a paediatric nurse and knew nothing of learning disability nursing, I didn't even know what learning disability meant – was it just being unable to learn? No, I found out and while going through the access to higher education course my journey changed, I decided that I had a lot to give and wanted to make a difference in people's lives that lived with everyday struggles and this led me to learning disability nursing. I wanted to make a difference, I wanted to enable people to live the lives they are entitled to live because while there have been massive advances in this field there is still so much more work to be done and I want a part in doing that. What the role gives is far more than just treating an illness; it's about holistic nursing and making changes to people's lives which to me is far more rewarding. Having reached the third year of my course I have seen the diversity of the role from community nursing, liaison nursing, private nursing, staff nurses, to advisory and rehabilitation nurses, but that's not all. If an individual has a passion to specialise there are so many fields open for them. Learning disability nurses make fantastic epilepsy specialist nurses, palliative care nurses, behavioural specialists and many more. Learning disability nursing really does open up many opportunities to make a difference. I have been fortunate to enjoy these varied roles and have gained so much from them. For me it's learning disability nursing all the way and I would never look back. I love all aspects of the role, I love the people I have the privilege of working with and most of all I love making a difference.'

Case study: Louise Drewett (third year student): 'The reason I chose learning disability (LD) nursing was because working with people with a learning disability was something I always wanted to do. This is not something that everyone can say but those that have chosen other areas of nursing have said they've gained a lot from their placement in LD areas and even changed fields. I get a lot out of supporting people with a learning disability through their life, supporting them to overcome difficulties, achieve their full potential and support them through health promotion and also support them through health worries. With LD nursing you support someone holistically and not just because of an illness they may have developed at any given time – you do not just give medication and then send the person on their way. You need to look at all the aspects of the person's life, whether that is their family life, their disability or current living accommodation, and implement the intervention which is most appropriate to enable the person to develop further. The thing I enjoy is working closely with people, finding out what they want and doing my best to support them with this. It is a challenge but I love that too.

I am not saying LD nursing is easy because it's not. You have to be able to think quickly and approach people differently due to their learning disability. You may need to use different methods of communication, body language and build relationships with people who may not trust you at first. LD nursing is diverse in terms of the needs of the people you will support and this is because everyone with a learning disability is unique. Support may be required within the community, within a residential setting, within an Assessment and Treatment Unit, within a secure setting, within hospital and within a prison. So LD nursing is not just about a health condition and the diversity is what makes LD nursing so rewarding and exciting; this is why I chose LD nursing and would not change my field for the world. I find LD nursing (even as student) rewarding, challenging, difficult and emotional but love everything I do.'

Case study: Tracy March (third year student): 'I am in my third and final year of study as a learning disability nurse at the University of Nottingham. Before I started my nursing course I had worked for the previous five and a half years in Health and Social care, predominantly with adults with learning disabilities. My final job was as a support worker within a Community Learning Disability Team and it was while in this role that I was encouraged by my peers to do my nursing education. There was never any doubt in my mind when choosing the learning disability field. There is so much out there career wise: community, assessment and treatment, forensics, residential, specialist school nurses, supported living and day services to name just a few. And then there are the people you work with who have such a wide and extensive variation of needs, personalities and disabilities.

I am passionate about those with learning disabilities having the same treatment as everyone else and hope to find a career in health facilitation. Learning disability nurses wear many hats and have to gain many skills, acquire new knowledge and face challenges constantly. We see our patients as a whole holistic package and it is this that spurs me on to qualify and hopefully make a difference to those I will meet in the future.'

Case study: Zoe Walters (second year student): 'When I first started the course in 2010 we were always asked why we chose to come into nursing. This question came with the same answer every time.... *'I want to make a difference'* ...it started to become a bit of a cliché and surprisingly made me smile the more I heard people say it... But when it got to the people on the route to become a learning disability nurse this changed, the answers varied and actually meant something, meant more. You will see amazing things, and meet some amazing people that will change the way you look at the world for the rest of your life.

Learning disability nursing is full of opportunities, a lifelong career that changes with you. As a friend, a colleague, and a nurse, you will be able to stand up and say I have made a difference and I will be able to do so for a long time! I enjoy every day of my training, I take advantage of every opportunity and most of all look forward to my future as a learning disability nurse.'

Case study: Abi Clay (second year student): 'I chose to do learning disability nursing at it has always been of interest to me and saw it as an opportunity to make a positive change in the lives of individuals with a learning disability.

From developing further into my training it becomes clearer day by day why I want to be a learning disability nurse. It allows me to be able to understand individuals who for most of their lives have been classed as 'different' but really are just as interesting and amazing as anyone else. It enabled me to realise that it is important that we give them the opportunity to live their lives to the full and support them in having the quality of life they deserve. From the experiences I have had and the people I have met during my training I couldn't wish for a better career and look forward to the future working as a learning disability nurse.'

The next account illustrates the type of challenging role that learning disability nurses can do:

Case study: Acute Learning Disability Liaison Nurse – Michelle Neal

'The role of the Acute Liaison Nurse is a relatively new one. It came about as a result of a number of reports which identified that people with LD do not always get equal access to healthcare. Mencap's *Death by Indifference* report, in 2007 which highlighted six cases of people with LD who died unnecessarily in NHS hospitals and the Local Authority Ombudsman *Six Lives* report which followed this, made a number of recommendations to try to address the "*significant and distressing failures*" experienced by people with learning disability while in hospital and help reduce the inadequate care and poor treatment that contributed towards the deaths of the six people in the report. One of these recommendations was that all acute hospitals should employ an Acute Learning Disability Liaison Nurse.

For me, because this was a brand new role, it has been an exciting opportunity to develop and establish a service which can provide specialist knowledge and expertise to assist people with learning disabilities and their carers achieve a positive experience and clinically appropriate outcomes while accessing acute hospital services. Achieving this has led to many challenges and has been a big learning curve both for myself and the many staff and partners I work with within the acute setting. However, seeing the positive outcomes and success stories for the people with learning disabilities and their carers make it all worthwhile!

I now have three main parts to my role:

Strategic: where I provide specialist knowledge and input into developing policies, practices and procedures for people with learning disabilities within the trust. This also involves designing and producing a vast and ongoing range of easy-to-read information and resources for patients, carers and staff; setting up a steering group to raise awareness of learning disabilities and devise care pathways for all clinical areas; assisting the trust to meet Care Quality Commission and commissioner's learning disabilities related targets and advising on learning disabilities related complaints and critical incidents.

Education: to deliver training to all acute hospital staff so that their knowledge of learning disabilities is enhanced in such a way that people with learning disabilities receive the best possible care and clinical outcomes. This also involves the provision of training to independent and private sector providers on my role and how I can support them and the people they care for. Education requirements also involve developing resource packs for all wards and departments, and ensuring reasonable adjustments are made for people with learning disabilities and their carers to make sure they can access services equitably.

Liaison: where I work directly with people with learning disabilities, their family, carers, community teams and staff within the hospital, to maximise a positive experience while receiving care from the hospital. This includes pre-admission assessments, care planning, pain assessment, discharge planning, safeguarding concerns and complaints to name but a few things. This part of the role is endless, but that is what makes it so exciting and why I never get bored!

Top tips

- It may be useful to get some experience of working with people with learning disabilities.

- Talk to people with learning disabilities and their families.

- Find out about what's available to people with learning disabilities in your area.

- Familiarise yourself with the current view of people with learning disabilities (media etc).

- Be clear about your reasons for wishing to work with this group.

Chapter summary

This chapter has given a brief overview of the role of the learning disability nurse. It is a unique and varied role that does not conform to the 'sickness' model of nursing. Instead it focuses on the whole person and every aspect of their life and learning disability nurses deal with people of all ages. It is challenging, stimulating, exciting and every day is different to the next. Learning disability nurses work in many areas in many roles and the qualification of a registered learning disability nurse will open many doors.

Key points

- The role of the learning disability nurse is a diverse role.

- Learning disability nurses do not work with 'sick' people; they work to empower the learning disabled person.

- Learning disability nurses work in many different environments, including NHS, private and charity organisations.

- Many of the roles for the learning disability nurse are specialist roles, in areas such epilepsy, challenging behaviour, forensic services, continence advice, acute liaison and health facilitation to name just a few.

Useful resources

Here are some websites that will help you understand a little more about the role of the learning disability nurse and those with learning disabilities:

http://learningdisabilitynurse.com

www.bild.org.uk

www.mencap.org.uk

www.challengingbehaviour.org.uk

www.autism.org.uk

www.downs-syndrome.org.uk

References

Bottomer, C (2004) Helping people look to new horizons. *Nursing Times* 22nd June 2004. Vol 100. No. 25. p. 54.

Department of Health (2001) *Valuing People: A New Strategy for Learning Disability for the 21st Century.* The Stationery Office.

Manthorpe, J *et al* Learning disability nursing: a multi-method study of education and practice. *Learning in Health and Social Care* 2004. Vol 3. No2 pp. 92-101.

Mencap (2007) *Death by Indifference.* Mencap: London

Michael, J (2008) *Healthcare For All: Report of the Independent Inquiry into Access to Healthcare for People with Learning Disabilities.* The Stationery Office.

Mitchell, D (2004) Learning disability nursing. *British Journal of Learning Disabilities.* No. 32. pp. 115-118.

Northway, R, Hutchinson, C and Kingdom, A eds (2006) *Shaping the Future: A Vision for Learning Disability Nursing.* London: UK Learning Disability Consultant Nurse Network.

Walmsley, J and Rolph, S (2001) The development of community care for people with learning disabilities 1913 to 1946. *Critical Social Policy.* 21(1) pp. 59-80.

Wright, D ed (1996) *From Idiocy to Mental Deficiency.* London: Routledge.

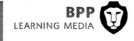

Chapter 5

Learning for practice and learning in practice

Gemma Stacey and
Anne Felton

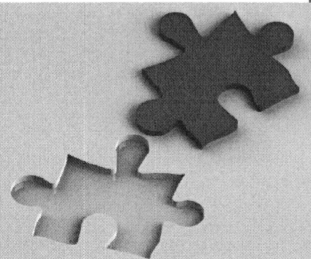

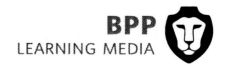

BPP
LEARNING MEDIA

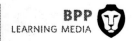

Introduction

Studying for a nursing qualification will require you to demonstrate competency in clinical skills, capability in justifying the way you deliver and manage care and confidence in communicating this with patients, colleagues and other healthcare professionals. There will be some skills that are common to all fields of nursing and some that will be more relevant to a specific practice area or setting and learning takes place both in a university setting and clinical practice areas. The following chapter will introduce you to learning methods and approaches commonly adopted in nurse education programmes. It will outline the prominent theories which underpin contemporary nurse education and the key areas of knowledge that you would be encouraged to develop in your journey from novice to capable practitioner.

Influential theories of learning in nurse education

The following will give you some insight into the theories of learning which will influence the way in which the nurse education programme you are considering is delivered. You may find that there is quite a bit of variation in the structure of the courses you are looking into, however the following brief descriptions will give you some idea of what you will be working towards.

Benner

The theory of learning proposed by Benner (1986) is named *From Novice to Expert: Excellence and Power in Clinical Nursing Practice*. It proposes that the learning journey encompasses five stages including novice, advanced beginner, competence, proficiency and expertise.

1.   In the novice stage the student learns through observation, instruction and demonstration. They are able to carry out a specific skill under supervision in a straightforward environment.

2.   The student develops to the advanced beginner stage when they are able to apply this learning in more intricate situations and adapt to some of the complexities presented to them in clinical practice.

3.   The competence stage is characterised by the student's ability to plan a sequence of tasks and provide justification for their course of action.

4.   This is developed further when students see a situation as a whole and are able to prioritise tasks. This stage is known as

proficiency and is defined by the student's ability to problem-solve and respond to situations outside of the norm.

5.   The final stage of expertise sees the practitioner as having the intuitive ability to understand the situation and act naturally without explicitly solving problems. They are also able to reflect on their intuition and see ways of improving practice.

From this description you can see how the student begins as slow, hesitant and perhaps somewhat anxious and develops to a fluid and intuitive practitioner who is able to problem-solve and provide sound rationale for the decisions that they make. Historically it has been assumed that expertise is acquired through experience and that these stages correlate to the number of years a person has been in practice. However more recently it has been acknowledged that this is not a linear process and that the rate at which expertise will be achieved is highly individual and context dependent (Gobet and Chassy, 2008). Additionally, the role of nurse has change significantly since the publication of this theory and there is now an expectation that newly qualified nurses should be able to demonstrate some of the attributes of an expert when they begin their career (Nursing and Midwifery Council, 2010).

Bondy

The evolving level of skill that you develop during your nurse education will be reflected in the expectations that your assessor in practice (mentor) and lecturers will have of you at different points in the course. The level of support and supervision expected to deliver care to service users and work as part of a multi-disciplinary team will decrease as you get towards the end of your course and prepare to graduate as a qualified nurse.

One of the frameworks commonly used to help students and mentors understand the level of performance of clinical skills required and whether these are being met has been developed by Kathleen Bondy. Bondy (1983) outlines that being competent at performing a skill involves three key areas:

* Professional standards: this criteria involves how knowledge is used to perform a skill safely, accurately and within the expectations of professional guidelines such as the Nursing and Midwifery Council (NMC) code (2008).

* Quality: essentially this aspect involves how well a skill is performed. This might include how equipment is used, how different aspects are co-ordinated and at later stages whether a student nurse is able to focus on the person alongside the

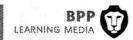

performance of a practical skill (such as giving an injection).

- Level of assistance needed to perform the skill: this relates to the amount of direction or prompting that may be given by a qualified member of staff to help you perform the skill.

Bondy (1983) also outlines the different levels at which skills may be carried out. These reflect your increasing levels of competency as you progress through the course. For example, when you first start you will be at an introductory level so would need more prompting, information and support from your mentor and may not perform the skill to the best quality. However, by the time that you are nearing the end of your course you should be practising at a more independent level performing a skill well and with minimal input from your mentor. Bondy's (1983) framework can help mentors and students make judgements about which level they are at and how they can develop to the next stage.

Areas of learning in nurse education

This section will introduce you to the key areas of learning which make up nurse education programmes. You will spend 50% of your programme in university and 50% in a number of different clinical practice environments. However, each of these areas of learning will span across both of these environments and you will be encouraged to consider how material covered in university links with your experiences in practice.

Clinical skills

Nursing practice involves an *'integration of thinking, feeling, doing, focusing on performance and judgement'* (Edmond, 2001). It is the 'doing' part of this that incorporates clinical skills. Nevertheless it is important to recognise that in carrying out a clinical skill effectively the other aspects that Edmond has outlined are essential. Often clinical skills are recognised as the 'psychomotor' skills that nurses might carry out such as giving an injection, taking a blood pressure and dressing a wound. However, clinical skills incorporate a much broader notion of the skills required to practise as a nurse and deliver high quality care. Abilities required in healthcare practice also include leading a team of people, making decisions and providing a reason for those decisions and identifying and responding to a person's non-verbal communication. Clinical skills will be an integral part of your nurse education and something you learn about within the practice setting and also in university.

Evidence-based practice

Evidence-based practice refers to the process by which healthcare professionals use different forms of evidence to inform their clinical judgements and decision-making. In this respect, evidence-based practice deals with the question of how nurses know that the care, support and treatment that they are providing to people using health and social care services is the best it possibly can be. Evidence-based practice has become a core feature of contemporary health services and is an expectation of the different health professions such as midwifery and medicine as well as being an approach that should underpin the development of national health policy and local guidelines for care.

There is debate as to what constitutes 'evidence' in respect of evidence-based practice. It is commonly understood to refer to research. This entails projects conducted by health professionals and qualified researchers to test out different treatments to examine the cause and consequences of health problems as well as explore service users' and professionals' experiences of ill health and treatment. These are published in professional journals. Gerrish (2010) highlights that research is only part of the way evidence-based practice is conceptualised and argues for a broader definition. Gerrish's (2010) perspective is reflected in other definitions of evidence-based practice which recognise that evidence can also incorporate the clinical experience and expertise of practitioners such as nurses as well as the preferences of service users and carers. This also recognises that there are some areas of healthcare practice where there is little or no research. It is also important to recognise that when research is carried out, there are many factors that can impact on the quality and relevance of that research and therefore research has to be applied to practice in a 'critical way'.

Values-based practice

The term 'values' is defined in the Oxford Dictionary in two ways. First, it is conceptualised as a set of principles or standards of behaviour. This definition is reflected in the ethical ideals of society or of a specific organisation like the NHS. These values are often externally prescribed by law, professional codes of conduct or organisational philosophies. Knowledge and understanding of the implications of these is essential for the maintenance of high standards of professional practice.

The second definition is stated as *'one's judgement of what is important in life'*. This description reflects the internal concept of values and relates to the person's own beliefs and morals which influence

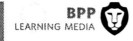

their attitudes and behaviour. Nurse education programmes are increasingly becoming aware of the need to consider how personal values influence the way in which nurses practise and respond to the healthcare environment. Research has demonstrated the conflicts that can exist between external and internal values which may have negative implications for the student nurse if left to resolve these issues in isolation (Stacey *et al*, 2010). Therefore there should be opportunity to consider these complexities in depth in order to also develop in the knowledge of ourselves which is known as self awareness.

Learning in university

'The mix of theory and practice makes the course really enjoyable and is great for those that either learn best in the classroom or by getting hands-on experience. The assignments although daunting at first are definitely manageable and there is lots of support where extra help is needed whether it be a quick question over email or a face-to-face tutorial.' **Samantha Thomas**

The following will give you a brief description of the types of teaching and learning approaches commonly adopted in nurse's education programmes when in the university setting.

Top tip

The degree to which these approaches are used will vary at different universities so it is important to consider how you prefer to learn when selecting a course.

Assess your skills

Use the questions below to think about your preferred learning style.

1. I learn best when information is

    a.   Presented to me
    b.   Given to me and I read it in my own time
    c.   Personally researched
    d.   Discussed in small groups

2. I enjoy working with others to learn

    a. Never
    b. Rarely
    c. Sometimes
    d. Always

3. I am motivated to learn

    a. In the classroom
    b. Independently
    c. Working in small groups
    d. All of the above

4. I see my lecturer as

    a. An expert to learn from
    b. A director of my learning
    c. A facilitator of my learning
    d. A partner in my learning

Use this information to consider the learning forums below and identify which would suit your preferred learning style.

Lectures

Lectures are usually the place in the curriculum where the key principles, concepts and knowledge base of the topic will be presented. You are usually in larger groups and it is advisable to be prepared to take notes. It is likely that you will be expected to engage in further reading to build upon the material presented to you in the lecture.

Problem-based learning or enquiry-based learning

This approach utilises case studies based on clinical scenarios which are used by the students to trigger their learning. This process is guided by a facilitator who supports the students to identify and research the knowledge skills and values which are relevant to the particular case.

Workshops

Workshop will usually involve a high level of student participation and group work. They may aim to explore the practical application of theoretical concepts or allow the student to practise a clinical skill.

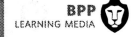

Simulation

Simulation is an approach which is adopted when learning a new or complex clinical skill. It will often take place in an environment which has been created to imitate the real practice setting and may use prosthetic models to allow you to practise in a controlled setting before applying a skill in the clinical area.

E learning

This approach will involve using the web to research areas which have been presented to you in other forums. It can also entail utilising packages which have been specially designed to meet specific learning outcomes. These can include things such completing online activities, watching video material or testing your knowledge with quizzes or mock exams.

Reflective forums

This type of learning approach usually involves working in small groups to consider your practice experiences in depth and explore the complex issues which it might trigger for you in a supportive way.

Student directed

Increasingly nursing programmes will expect you to engage in your own learning outside of the classroom environment. This will be guided by the tutor and will be your opportunity to explore the content of the module in more depth through the consideration of different sources of evidence and alternative views.

Academic expectations

The academic level you will be expected to work at will depend on the structure and type of course you choose. This could be at degree level or masters level. Most courses are incremental in terms of academic expectations and start by requiring you to submit different types of assessments which are marked against specific criteria. The complexity of the assessment and marking criteria will change as the course progresses and the expectations become higher.

The key elements that you are judged by in a nursing programme are your ability to present a well-structured and articulate piece of work which shows evidence of critical discussion and application of theory to practice. The depth of critical discussion is expected to develop as the course progresses and you become confident in appraising the research literature available, comparing with your observations of practice and making sound judgments based on these factors. Alternatively assessment will be examining your level of knowledge in an exam setting which again will normally increase from factual understanding to clinical application.

You are not expected to become an expert in every element of nursing within your chosen field. However, the academic assessments are intended to equip you with the skills to know how to learn, respond confidently to the unfamiliar, question the status quo and adapt to change. It is these qualities that are viewed as attributes of graduate nurses and essential for meeting the demands of the future face of nursing.

Top tip

The following text will give a more detailed in sight into the academic expectations of a nursing programme and will help you make sense of what we mean by being 'critical'.

Price, B and Harrington A (2010) *Critical Thinking and Writing for Nursing Students*. Exeter: Learning Matters Ltd.

Learning in practice

Half of all time in nurse education is spent in health and social care settings. Nursing students therefore get the opportunity to work with service users and carers and different healthcare professions in the environment where care is delivered. This could involve working on the ward in a hospital, visiting service users in their own homes, working in residential homes, high secure hospitals or hospices to give a few examples. This will include being placed in organisations run by the NHS, voluntary organisations and charities alongside private healthcare providers. The range of areas or settings that you gain experience of will depend on what field of practice you have chosen and how the university where you are studying has structured these practice experiences. Learning in practice in contemporary nurse education is designed so that you get to experience care in a number of different settings that include in-patient areas (such as hospitals) and community areas (such as visiting people in their own homes).

When you are working in those settings your role as a student nurse is clearly defined. This means that you contribute to care while in the setting but are not classed as a member of staff, so that you have the opportunity to focus on your learning and on developing your skills. In order to enable you to do this in every placement you will be allocated a 'mentor'.

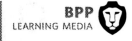

'I thoroughly enjoy when the time comes to go into practice as a student nurse. I feel the university helps in ensuring you get a varied amount of placements in different fields of nursing which helps you find things you enjoy and others you don't. I find the mentors in practice great; they really do go out of their way to help you in furthering your knowledge in practical work and theory.' **Kirsty Fletton**

Mentor

A mentor is a qualified member of nursing staff whose role it is to support and assess pre-registration student nurses. In order to act as a mentor this member of staff will have undertaken additional training in teaching and learning strategies and attended regular updates about nurse education. They will be responsible for ensuring you have the relevant information when you start your placement, help you set goals for your learning and identify how you will work towards your goals in that setting. They will also assess your performance and whether you have achieved specific skills and knowledge to the required standard. These are known as competencies. They undertake this role in addition to the work they conduct as a nurse.

Competencies

The Nursing and Midwifery Council define competence as an *'overarching set of knowledge, skills and attitudes required to practise safely and effectively without direct supervision'* (NMC, 2010). The NMC has broken this down into a number of distinct areas that nursing students are required to demonstrate competence in at different levels during their practice experiences. These cover four domains:

- Professional values
- Communication and interpersonal skills
- Nursing practice and decision-making
- Leadership, management and team working

Your university will provide you with more specific detail regarding skills for each area in a practice document. During your time in clinical settings you will be working towards achieving these competencies and your mentor will assess your performance against each one.

Following some concerns about the level of skill that newly qualified nurses were graduating with, the NMC identified a number of *'essential skills'* that student nurses needed to be assessed against at particular points in their education. Students are assessed to check they are competent in these particular areas in the practice setting. There are some differences in what is defined as an essential skill in each field (adult, mental health, child or learning disabilities), though they cover these areas:

- Care, compassion and communication
- Organisational aspects of care
- Infection prevention and control
- Nutrition and fluid management
- Medicines management

'Looking back, I would now say to any student that while it's ok to be nervous about starting a placement there is no need to be really scared or worried about it. Every placement I've been on (and I'm now on my seventh) whether it be acute or community based have been very welcoming and helpful. Mentors try their best to have you work with them on all of their shifts and so you will probably find that you end up working with your mentor a lot more than the required 40% of your placement time. I have only ever had one issue on placement where I felt I could not talk to my mentor however this was dealt with quickly and positively with the ward sister. All of my placement experiences have been nothing but positive. It is amazing looking back just how nervous I was in the first year. I now think nothing of going into a new placement area and introducing myself and explaining what skills and experiences I have had so far.' **Samantha Thomas**

Expectations during practice experiences

Hours

While working in the practice setting, students work full-time hours and are expected to follow the pattern of shifts within that particular area. These will clearly differ depending on the setting but many areas are staffed 24 hours a day by nurses. This may involve working early shifts, starting around 7.00am and finishing early afternoon, late shifts starting at lunchtime and finishing around 9.00pm and night shifts covering the night-time hours. Several areas work 12-hour shifts but have more days off. There are also areas, particularly in the community or clinics that work traditional office hours during the day. Universities and healthcare areas will have policies in place that help to protect students and ensure that they have a fair range of shift patterns in one practice experience. However, it's important that you give thought to the implications of shift work during your education for other areas of your life. Consideration should be given to how the practicalities of this might be managed, for example transport and making sure that you have the support at home to commit to working these hours.

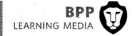

Conduct

Throughout your nurse education and your future career, there are guidelines that you will be expected to practise within. Generally, these guidelines are produced by the NMC (NMC, 2008), though universities may have also developed further documents to outline their expectations of nursing students. These identify the conduct expected of nurses and cover areas such as how you relate to other people, how you behave and how you manage information. The role of these guidelines is both about protecting the public and keeping up the high standards of the nursing profession.

The NMC code of professional conduct (2008) outlines the standards expected of nurses that include:

- Respecting the patient as an individual
- Protecting confidential information
- Co-operating with others

Top tip

Become familiar with the NMC guidelines in preparation for your interview or include reference to this in your personal statement. These are available at www.nmc-uk.org/.

It is important to remember that for a job such as nursing, your conduct both within university and outside of working hours is also really important. In this respect for example, bullying on Facebook, being derogatory about service users and claiming other people's academic work as your own are examples of poor conduct that could have implications for your future career as a nurse. As highlighted above, while in healthcare settings, although student nurses are not members of staff, there are clear expectations about conduct, appearance and performance.

Nurses undergoing their pre-registration education will be expected to adopt a professional approach. This professionalism is demonstrated in many ways and will be an area that you cover in the classroom before going out into healthcare settings.

Assessment

Types of assessment

The following descriptions will give you some insight into the ways you might be assessed when completing a nursing programme. Again, different universities favour different approaches to assessment, so it is a good idea to enquire about this in order to find the right type of course for you. However, it is good practice to have a variety of assessment approaches within a programme, so it is likely that most courses will encompass a mixture of the following.

Exams

As you will be aware from your previous studies, exams are assessments which are carried out in a controlled environment where you are not able to confer with your peers or consult other sources. They can comprise a series of multiple choice questions, short answer questions or essays and are used to test specific knowledge.

Objective Structured Clinical Examinations (OSCEs) or practical exams

OSCEs are used to assess competence in clinical skills in a simulated environment. You will be watched undertaking the task by an examiner and marked against predefined criteria.

Essays

Essays in nursing programmes usually involve a written demonstration of how you have linked relevant theory to your practice, explored the research evidence pertinent to the topic and reflected upon your professional development. They will vary in length and focus, but should always include critical discussion of the material presented.

Presentations

This approach to assessment will involve the verbal presentation of your work / assignment. You may be also required to incorporate visual aids such as PowerPoint and both the presentation style and content will be considered as part of the assessment process.

Posters

Poster presentations require you to convey material in a succinct and interesting way. You may be asked to present the content of your poster verbally as part of the assessment, however it should be able to stand alone as a clear representation of the research, theory and practical application of the topic.

Extended projects / dissertations

Extended projects or dissertations are longer pieces of work which may involve carrying out a piece of research, implementing a development

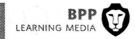

in practice or conducting an in-depth review of literature. You will usually be assigned a supervisor who will support you in identifying your topic, planning your work and will feed back on its development and direction throughout the process.

Progression points

Throughout the programme there will be specific points where your progress will be reviewed in order to ensure you are meeting the criteria which is set by the university and the Nursing and Midwifery Council. These are known as progression points and include consideration of the following:

- Achievement of practice competencies at the required level
- Achievement of academic credits at the required level
- Attendance at or completion of mandatory materials

In order for you to continue on the programme, you must have met all of these requirements by the progression points, unless you have specific circumstances which have prevented you from doing so. These are commonly at the end of Year 1 and Year 3 for a three-year BSc course.

Student support

This chapter has highlighted the range of experiences that you undertake during nurse education in addition to providing some insight into the teaching and assessments structures, as well as the expectations on student nurses as emerging professionals. This highlights that nursing education is a rich and rewarding experience, but also a demanding one. During your course there are many resources available to support you in this journey. A range of student services are available, often run in partnership with students unions, providing support and information regarding practical issues such as housing and finances. Academic support services or tutors are able to provide students with additional input in developing study skills and in helping those students who may have additional learning needs such as dyslexia. During your education, you will also have a tutor or supervisor who will work with you during the whole of the course. They have a pastoral role so can help you make the most of your course, but also provide support and as well as putting you in touch with other sources of help if you have health or personal problems that impact on your studies. Many universities have also developed other ways of supporting students such as introducing junior and senior students to offer peer support and advice. This might be an area you want to explore when making choices about where to study.

Case study

The following example gives a brief outline of the early part of one first year student's course.

Katie started at a school of healthcare studies in September. Before starting her course Katie was invited to a pre-course day where she had the opportunity to meet some of the staff and other students she would be studying with. Naturally Katie was nervous about her course but on the first day Katie met her personal tutor. This was important for Katie as she had a few questions about her timetable and what support she would get with her dyslexia that her personal tutor could answer for her, and they continued to meet every couple of months during Katie's first year.

Katie's course started with an introduction to many of the practical issues of being a university nursing student. Katie had two and a half months before her first placement and in this time attended lectures on, amongst other topics, the anatomy and physiology of the cardiovascular system, and the history of nursing and policy developments in healthcare. She is currently part of a seminar study group with other students studying adult nursing. In this group they are working through a case study of 'the Kleine family', where each week they are given some information about changes in the family's health or social circumstances by their group facilitator; they then have to research the topic and discuss it as a group the following week. However, Katie's favourite sessions as they are 'hands on' are the clinical skills ones where they have so far learned about taking a blood pressure, administering medication and communicating with people.

Katie is excited but nervous about her first placement which is on a stroke rehabilitation ward in a community hospital. The ward have sent Katie an induction pack and she has spoken to the ward on the phone to find out about her first shifts and the uniform policy. When she finishes the placement and after her holiday Katie has to hand in her first assignment, which is an essay on a skill that she has carried out on her placement. Katie is planning to book a tutorial with her module lecturer about this nearer the time. She has had a busy first few weeks on the course, but Katie is really looking forward to starting on the ward.

You might want to think about what learning approaches are described here and also the support strategies that are mentioned in the description of the early part of Katie's course.

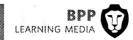

Chapter summary

This chapter has described the ways in which you would be learning for practice and learning in practice when undertaking a nurse education programme. The ways in which this is interpreted and implemented will vary across the different universities, so it is important to identify the structure and format of the courses that you are considering. The information here should help you to ask the right questions to ensure you make the decision which best fits with your personal learning style and requirements. It is evident that nurse education is demanding and requires a great deal of commitment. It is important therefore to have a good awareness of what would be expected of you in terms of both practical and academic obligations.

Key points

- It is important to consider the structure and format of the courses that you are considering.
- Nurse education programmes include 50% learning in the university and 50% in the clinical environment.

Useful resources

NMC website
www.nmc-uk.org/

Open University Study Support pages
http://www.open.ac.uk/skillsforstudy/develop-effective-study-strategies.php

Levett-Jones, T and Bourgeois, S (2009) *The Clinical Placement: A Nursing Survival Guide.* London: Ballier Tindall.

Price, B and Harrington A (2010) *Critical Thinking and Writing for Nursing Students.* Exeter: Learning Matters Ltd.

References

Benner, P (1984) *From Novice to Expert: Excellence and Power in Clinical Nursing Practice*. Menlo Park, CA: Addison-Wesley.

Bondy, K. Criterion referenced definitions for rating scales in clinical evaluation. *The Journal of Nurse Education* 1983; 22(9): 376-82.

Edmond, C. A new paradigm for practice education. *Nurse Education Today* 2001: 21: 251-9.

Gerrish, K (2010) 'Evidence based practice' In Gerrish, K, Lacey, A eds. *The Research Process in Nursing*. 6th edition. Chichester: Wiley-Blackwell.

Gobet, F and Chassy, P. (2008) Towards an alternative to Benner's theory of expert intuition in nursing: A discussion paper. *International Journal of Nursing Studies*. 45(1) 129-139.

Nursing and Midwifery Council (2008) *The Code: Standards of Conduct, Performance, and Ethics for Nurses and Midwives*. London: NMC.

Nursing and Midwifery Council (2010) *Standards for Pre-registration Nursing Education*. London: NMC.

Nursing and Midwifery Council (2010) *Standards for Pre-registration Education. Explanation of terms*. [Online] Available at http://standards.nmcuk.org/PreRegNursing/statutory/explanation/Pages/explanation-of-terms.aspx [Accessed October 2011].

Stacey G, Johnston, K, Stickley, T and Diamond, B. How do nurses cope when values and practice conflict? *Nursing Times* 2010: 107(5): 20-23.

Unison (2004) *Oxford Dictionary of Nursing*. Oxford: Oxford University Press.

Chapter 6

Choosing the right course for you and making a successful application to university

Gail Mitchel

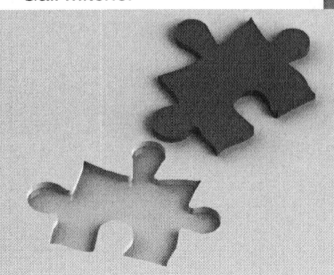

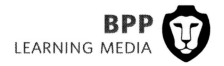

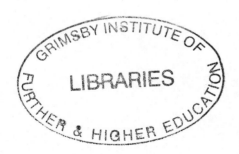

BPP
LEARNING MEDIA

Introduction

So you have decided that nursing is the career for you and see your future in a profession that is more than 'just a job'. You have identified that you want to do something interesting, something that makes the best use of your skills and qualities, involves working as part of a team and enables you to continue to learn and develop throughout your career. Above all perhaps, you want a career that centres on helping people.

That you are reading this book suggests you have already started on the road to success; it might seem obvious, but investigating the options in tandem with an honest assessment of your own motivations and qualities increases the likelihood that you will make a successful application, enjoy your course, achieve your degree in nursing and go on to a long, happy and productive career as a nurse.

Having made the decision that this is the right career for you, this chapter is about helping you to make those first formal steps towards securing a place on a nursing degree course at the right university for you. It will help you to plan a course of action aimed at identifying the university and course that best suits you. Key features of recruitment and selection methods will be highlighted so that you understand the process. Perhaps most importantly, the chapter aims to give you ideas about how you can increase your chances of a successful application.

The chapter is broken down into three broad sections with related sub-sections that reflect the steps that you will be making as you pursue your ambition.

- Choosing a university and course
- Understanding the application process
- Improving your chances of securing a place at your university of choice

Choosing a university and course

Let's start this section by hearing from two students currently studying for degrees in Adult nursing:

Sam says: *'When I applied to study nursing I knew that there was only one place I wanted to study. When I applied to the course I did so because of what I had seen of the nursing staff that cared for my relative when they were in hospital for a long period of time, therefore*

> *I wanted to be working alongside nursing staff I knew to be of a good professional standard. That relative was still unwell when I applied and they still needed my support, therefore I had to stay close to them, which was another reason I applied. In addition, I knew this university had a good reputation for their nursing course so I was happy with limiting my choice to just the one academic institution.'*

Sam was very clear about her priorities in choosing to apply to just one university.

Martelle approached things a little differently. She reports:

> 'As I consider myself to have a caring and compassionate nature, I somehow think that the choice to study nursing was made for me and therefore I'm merely walking in my destiny. However, difficulty arose when deciding which university to go to and which of the many nursing courses to study. I had already made the decision that I wanted to study away from home, as I think it is better preparation for the real world. I also wanted to be on a course that was academically challenging without neglecting the practical essentials of clinical nursing practice. I searched for the possibility of studying abroad during the course and also, which universities were high up in the rankings. Collectively, these reasons led me to my final choice'.

Both Sam and Martelle, in their different ways, decided what was important to them in making an application for a nursing degree and this is what influenced them in their choice of university course. This is an essential early stage for you and you should think about what is going to be important for **you** in choosing a university. Your first step then is to identify priorities that will influence your choice of where to study.

Background research and drawing up a shortlist

At this point you are ready to do some preliminary research, for example looking at the University and College Admissions Service (UCAS) website (www.ucas.ac.uk) to identify which universities provide nursing degrees in the geographical areas you are interested in. From this initial search, you may want to draw up a 'long list' of potential universities that seem to fit your requirements. You can then begin to focus your search and investigate in more depth; your aim now should be to narrow down your choices to the maximum of five permitted by the application system (more information on this later in the chapter).

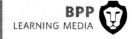

Progressing from your long list to a final shortlist will take time and energy when you are busy with other things in your life (examinations, jobs, family life, etc) but it is well worth the effort to increase your chances of pinpointing the right environment for your nursing studies.

There are lots of resources you can use to get the information you need – many are at your fingertips if you have access to the internet.

Ideas of where to look include:

- University prospectuses – both printed and online versions
- UCAS website – www.ucas.ac.uk
- Newspaper supplements – guides to university courses are produced annually and often include 'league tables'. To be really helpful to you, it is important these tables make very clear what elements are being judged so look out for explanations of their criteria.
- Independent websites that collate information about universities and courses, eg www.thecompleteuniversityguide.co.uk

Additionally, you can get a sense of what current students think about their university and course by accessing the results of the National Student Survey. This survey of final year students is conducted annually in all Higher Education Institutions (HEIs) in England, Wales and Northern Ireland. Some Scottish universities also participate. The results can be found at the Unistats website – http://unistats.direct.gov.uk. It is important to emphasise that while universities can and do encourage their students to participate, the survey itself is conducted by an independent organisation and completed anonymously by final year students. You may feel that this promotes the likelihood that students have made an honest assessment but you can only see a statistical breakdown of the data – there are no qualitative comments from the students.

A more personalised account of student experience can be found on social networking websites and other online student communities. It is beyond the remit of this chapter to make recommendations, however you are strongly advised to check out the purpose of the website and examine their policy for making complaints and removing inappropriate content. It is important to establish that you are using a safe and trustworthy source and to remain objective when you are assessing content of websites.

Visiting your shortlisted universities

While it is relatively straightforward to find information about universities and courses and also get an impression of what other people think, there is no substitute for getting a real feel of a place for yourself. This means capitalising on opportunities to visit, look around and, most importantly, talking with people at the university.

Universities know how important it is that you make the right choice, indeed it is in their interests to ensure that 'wrong university or course choice' is not a reason for students dropping out of university (Taylor, 2005; Glogowska, Young and Lockyer 2007; Waters, 2010). Thus they provide a range of opportunities to visit, including as 'open days'. Most universities hold these events on a number of dates in the year – particularly at the key points when they know that prospective students are researching their options. Great opportunities are presented to have a really good look around and to chat with academic staff and current students in the nursing department. You will probably have the chance to attend presentations about various aspects of the course and student life at the university. They are often very busy events with lots of like-minded people visiting which can really help you focus and look forward to joining the academic community. However, it can be easy to get carried away with the excitement and 'buzz' of the event and then find you have come away without having your questions answered. It is a good idea to have a plan of action for the day – where do you want to visit? Who do you want to talk to? – and to draw up a list of questions you would like answering.

Universities often supplement their open days with other opportunities to visit eg self-guided tours of the campus or perhaps a drop-in day when the nursing department will be open to visitors for a limited period of time. These events may be a little less hectic than an open event and can enable you to get an idea of how the university or department operates on an ordinary working day.

You may already have a clear idea of what you want to find out when you visit, although it is not uncommon to feel a little uncertain as to what you should be looking for or the questions you should be asking at this stage. Please be assured you will get better at working out what is important for you as you undertake more visits and become more familiar with the process but you might want to consider the following ideas to get you started.

Case study: Useful questions

To give you some pointers for drawing up your list of questions, a group of nursing students were asked what they had wanted to find out (or what, on reflection, they now think they should have found out!) when they were making their own choices. Here are some of their ideas:

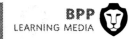

Questions about the university – location, geographical relationship of the nursing department to other departments

- Is it in a hospital? Is it close to the main university campus?
- What are the public transport links like?
- Is accommodation available and where? Will I be sharing with other nursing students or is there an opportunity to share with students from different courses?

Questions about the nursing department

- How big is it? How many undergraduate students?
- How many lecturers are involved in teaching on the undergraduate programmes?
- Does it have more than one centre and are students expected to travel for lectures?
- What are the facilities like? Are there any spaces specifically for learning skills and what equipment is available to help with this?
- Does the department offer other programmes eg post graduate degrees, specialist degrees in health-related areas? (Students felt that these can be important in planning for the future.)
- How many staff are involved in doing research and how is the department rated for its research? (Students felt proud to be at a university that is amongst the top in the country for research and recognised the importance of reputation, but also recognised how research underpins the teaching that undergraduate nurses receive.)

Questions about course detail

- How is the course structured? What subjects will I learn and how will my learning be assessed?
- How many hours study am I expected to complete each week? How much contact time will I have with lecturers?
- How many students will there be in a class? Are there are opportunities to learn with other healthcare students such as pharmacy, medical and physiotherapy students?

Questions about practice placements

- When will I be in practice? What range of placements is available?
- What travel is involved to placements and is there any financial support for this?

- How many hours will I work in placement?

- Is there any choice of practice placements? Are there any opportunities to experience practice in a different geographical area or to gain experience in a different country eg an 'elective' or exchange placement?

Questions about progression

- How many graduates go straight into employment and what kinds of jobs do they get and where?

Questions about support

- How much contact can students expect to receive from a personal tutor?

- Are there arrangements to support students when they first go into practice?

- What support is available for students with a disability?

- What happens if a student is struggling with any aspect of their course or something in their personal life that affects their studies?

This section has given you some ideas about your first step – how to ensure you are making an informed choice when selecting your university course. We will now go to the next stage – making your application and making sure it a successful one.

Understanding the application process

Applications for nursing degrees in the United Kingdom are managed by the University and College Admissions Service (UCAS). You may already have had information about this organisation from your school or college. Whether this is the case or you are new to this system, it is highly recommended you spend some time familiarising yourself with the process and there is excellent information available under the 'student' tab on the UCAS website www.ucas.ac.uk.

University admissions teams do find there are commonly held misconceptions about the applications process so it is worth summarising and perhaps clarifying some key aspects.

- You can choose to apply for **up to** five courses. This might be five different universities although it is also possible you will want to apply for more than one course at a particular university. As an example, Nottingham University offers a three-year BSc in Nursing and a four-year undergraduate Master of Nursing

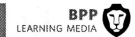

Science both leading to registration as a nurse; these are two separate choices.

Remember, you don't have to select five, but you do need to decide what your priorities are – you may know you want to study and live in a large city and at this stage you don't mind which one or, like Sam who we heard from earlier, personal circumstances or preferences mean you wish to apply to only one university.

This is an important decision – you will want to give yourself the best possible chance of gaining a place, but there is little point expending time and energy on applications for universities you know are not going to suit your needs.

- Universities only know what course(s) you have applied to at their institution, they don't know where else you may consider. This often surprises applicants who perhaps worry that a particular university will be unhappy because a student has applied elsewhere and that this will be a negative influence on their decision to make you an offer – in fact you're other choices are 'invisible'.

Top tip

You may be unsure what field of nursing you are interested in and decide to apply for more than one hoping you will be successful with at least one. Nothing in the UCAS process prevents you from doing this, although specific universities may have a policy that you should only apply for one field. Check this out with your chosen universities and take it into account (see also later section about personal statements).

- Once you have applied to UCAS, your application goes to all your chosen universities at the same time ie your application is considered simultaneously by all the institutions.

- All universities will work to the same timescales and deadlines set by UCAS, the date when decisions must be made for those who made an application by the initial closing date of 15th January (for 2013 applications). However, within these parameters there may be considerable variability in each institution's timetable. You should not worry if universities respond at different times; it does not mean, for example, that because you have not heard about an interview day at a particular university, you are low down in a preference list of applicants. You can get information about timescales from the admissions department of your chosen university either from their website or you can contact them by phone or email.

- After the selection process is completed (once all the selection events have been held), the university will decide on your application. This might be an offer of a place and this offer would be conditional if you need to pass examinations at a particular grade. Universities can reject your application if they do not consider you suitable for their course. This may happen when they make an initial assessment of your application form or following an interview / selection day. If this is the case, it is acceptable to ask for feedback to help you to strengthen any future applications.

- You are able to 'hold' two offers from your chosen courses / universities. One of these might be your first choice ie your 'firm' offer, but you may also want to keep a reserve option – an 'insurance' choice. Typically your insurance choice is a reserve place you can take up if you are unable to meet the conditions of your firm offer, generally because you don't achieve the examination grades you needed.

  Take your time in accepting offers; don't take the first one that comes your way (unless you are absolutely certain it is what you want) but make sure that you weigh up all offers once you have completed all of your interviews / selection days.

- If you accept an offer – whether as firm or insurance – this is then binding on the university and they cannot normally withdraw this unless there are additional professional conditions associated with health or criminal activity that have not been met (see more about this in the later section on professional perspectives).

- Final confirmation of conditional offers is made immediately after examination results are published in August.

You may have heard of other schemes that UCAS administer such as 'Extra' and 'Clearing'. These are aimed at matching vacancies on courses with suitable applicants who are searching for a place. There is insufficient space here to go into detail about these routes, but you are strongly advised to read about them on the UCAS website and to discuss the implications for you with your school / college or other educational advisor. University admissions departments should also be able to give you information about whether they will be participating in these schemes.

Having ensured that you are well informed about the application process and know which universities you are interested in, let's move to the next stage – making a successful application.

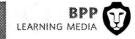

Improving your chances of securing a place at your university of choice

What are universities looking for in potential nursing students?

Let's start at the end here! Think about the kind of knowledge, skills, values and characteristics you might expect of a Registered Nurse – your background research and the other chapters in this book should help you build up a picture of what this person might look like. You may have been able to observe nurses at work during your work experience or perhaps from your own encounters with health services.

Obviously the course is designed to enable you to meet the standard required to join the professional register of nurses in three or four years (depending on the type of degree), but it is important that students admitted to nursing degrees possess **personal and ethical attributes** that will enable them to be successful in their course and ultimately to thrive in a career in nursing. This potential is what admissions teams will be looking for in your application.

Clearly you need the **intellectual capacity** to follow an academically challenging and demanding degree programme. Educational entry requirements will be set and must be attained but it is important not to just think of these as a hurdle to be cleared to achieve your ambition, but also as a way of preparing you for higher education – developing the skills and knowledge you need to be an independent learner and to be able to capitalise on all of the learning experiences that will come your way once on the course. To be successful as a nursing student you should be **open** to experiences, **curious** about life and **ready to explore** new ideas and concepts. Underestimating the commitment to study is a factor frequently cited for students not completing the course (O'Donnell, 2011; Cameron, Roxburgh, Taylor and Lauder, 2011).

This intellectual capacity also complements the qualities of **compassion** and **care** for others. These qualities are often difficult to discern, but you may want to ask yourself whether you are able to focus on the needs of others and, crucially, do you understand that it might not be enough to recognise somebody needs your help but you must also be able to recognise your ability to act on those needs. Remember, the word 'nursing' is a verb as well as a noun – it requires **action** on the part of the practitioner.

In order to do this, you will need to show some diverse skills such as the ability to communicate effectively with a range of different people – this means listening as well as verbal skills. High levels of literacy and confidence in your ability with numbers are perhaps more tangible skills and are essential if you are to succeed as a nursing student.

A number of other key personal attributes will be assessed. Qualities such as **conscientiousness** (can you take responsibility for yourself? Are you self-disciplined? Well organised?) and **emotional** stability (can you cope with stressful situations? Are you resilient when things don't go quite as expected?) have been identified as indicators of success in nursing students (Mclaughlin, Moutray and Muldoon, 2008).

Top tip

All of this might sound rather demanding and somewhat daunting, but please remember that admissions teams are not aiming to recruit fully-fledged graduate nurses but are looking for applicants who can show their potential to benefit from undertaking a nursing degree.

Professional perspectives

Nursing, like midwifery, differs from most other university courses in that there are additional demands apart from those set by the university and UCAS. The organisation that regulates nurses and midwives, the Nursing and Midwifery Council (NMC), specifies a number of criteria that must be met in selecting and admitting students for nursing courses. The overarching principle is one of creating an open and fair system that also ensures that students admitted to the course are of good health and good character. This is part of the statutory responsibility of the NMC in safeguarding the health and wellbeing of the public and is aimed at upholding the reputation of nurses as honest and trustworthy professionals.

Top tip

You can find more information about what it means to be of good character and good health on the NMC website at www.nmc-uk.org. You might also find it interesting and informative to read the guidance on professional conduct for nursing students (see resource section). Reading this guidance will help you think through what it means to be a student nurse from a professional perspective and would be good preparation for an interview or selection day.

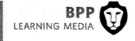

How universities assess your application – the importance of the personal statement

The UCAS personal statement is your first opportunity to introduce yourself formally to the universities you are interested in and to begin to show that you have the potential discussed earlier.

You will know from reviewing UCAS guidance that you have a limited number of words in which to communicate your reasons for choosing a nursing degree and your readiness to study nursing at university. You must make the most of this opportunity by staying focused and making each word and every sentence count. There is no space for irrelevant material or 'waffle'!

There is lots of advice and guidance available about writing your statement from your educational advisors and the UCAS website. Many universities also offer information on their web pages. You should read / listen to this advice carefully.

A nursing admissions team will be looking for a number of key aspects in your statement. These include:

- A professional approach to presentation. The statement must be written in good English, free of spelling and typographical errors. Keep it simple and try to avoid using complicated words or phrases because you think they sound good.

- Your statement should reflect **you** and your personality, not an idealised version of a student you have seen or read about on a website about applications.

- Your statement shows what you have experienced and achieved in life so far and, crucially, relates this to the course and field you are applying for. For example, you may be applying for child nursing and want to highlight that you held down a baby-sitting job or volunteered in a play scheme. This is good experience, but a strong application will show what you learned from those experiences and how the skills / knowledge gained might relate and apply to the role of a child nurse.

- Your statement should show you have insight into nursing in the field you are applying for. There is a potential difficulty here if you decided to apply for more than one field (or perhaps for different disciplines such as midwifery and nursing). In trying to show your understanding of more than one area, there is a real risk that you will dilute your personal statement which might have a detrimental effect on your chances of getting a place if courses are over-subscribed.

A word about work experience

In deciding that nursing is for you, it would be anticipated that you have gained experience that has demonstrated that you have the attributes that make a good nurse. Ideally, this experience would be in a health (or care) related setting. However, please note that this does not have to be in a hospital. Admissions teams are aware that it can be difficult to gain work experience (whether voluntary or paid) in such a setting, but will usually be looking for evidence of your understanding of nursing work and any relevant transferrable skills you have gained from your own work or life experience – eg working as a member of a team, taking responsibility for others and dealing with challenging situations.

Admissions teams will assess each UCAS application and personal statement using the criteria set for their particular course. Those applicants who meet the criteria at the required level will progress to the next stage of selection. Clearly you need to be on course to meet the academic requirements (or have previously attained these) but it is the **evidence** in your personal statement that can make the difference between being rejected at this stage or progressing towards your goal of gaining a place.

So take your time, do your research – and aim to make a great **personal** statement.

The next stage – selection for a place

Universities will vary in the methods they use to select students for their nursing course. However, the NMC require every HEI to ensure the selection process always includes 'face-to-face engagement' (NMC, 2008). This means that unlike many other degree subjects, you cannot be offered a place without attending the university for an interview or other type of selection event.

There is also a requirement that partner 'service' organisations are involved in the process. Thus both academic and NHS staff contribute to the selection of students for courses. Universities are also encouraged to involve 'lay' people (those who aren't nurses) in selection activities, and in particular, people who are users of health services and their carers.

You can see from this that you must expect to meet with, and be assessed by, a variety of people as part of your selection for your chosen course.

Types of selection methods include:

- Face-to-face interviews
- Group interviews

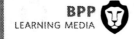

- Group problem-solving exercises
- Test in literacy and numeracy

These may be used individually or in combination. The principle underpinning all of these is that applicants do not just say what knowledge or skills they possess, they must **demonstrate** this. So, it is not enough to say that you have effective communication skills – you must show you have these skills in a new situation such as an interview or problem-solving exercise. Similarly, there is no point in saying you have a passion for nursing if you don't show you have done something to find out what nurses do or the kinds of health issues that might be of concern in your chosen field.

Again, this may sound a little daunting, but your interviewers / assessors will understand this and try to put you at ease. Your aim is to prevent any nervousness from spoiling your opportunity to show what you can do and demonstrate why you should be awarded a place.

Clearly, it is essential for you to find out what selection method is used by the university course you are applying for; there will often be useful information about how to get ready for the day on the university or departmental web page.

Whatever method is used, you need to spend time in preparation. This will include thinking through different elements, from the practicalities – how you are going to get there on time and what you might wear on the day for example – through to fine detail, making sure that you know what you have written in your personal statement and, importantly, can expand on this in an interview or group discussion.

It is also useful preparation to do some reading and reflecting on any health issues that are in the news – this shows interviewers / assessors that you are interested in some of the broader issues that have an impact on the health of individuals, families and communities and can think about how these might relate to the role of the nurse.

Top tip

There are a number of excellent sources of information to help and some useful websites are listed in the resources section at the end of the chapter. You can also read current copies of professional journals such as the *Nursing Times* and *Nursing Standard* that are available from major newsagents. These journals run interesting news stories and you often won't need specialist knowledge to understand them.

You will see the key word in all of this is 'preparation'. Whatever the format of the day, preparation gives you the confidence to really show assessors you have taken the selection process seriously and you have the skills and qualities they are looking for in a nursing degree student.

If you have done the preparation, you have given yourself the best chance of securing a place, even if you have never experienced an interview situation before.

> **Emma, a second year student reflecting on her interview experiences, reports:**
>
> *'The interviews were definitely daunting and you never know what is coming on the day. I prepared some answers to questions I thought I would get asked then forgot them all! But I just took time to think through everything I was asked. Ultimately it's important to be yourself and show them why you would make a good nurse. Nurses are often thrown into tricky situations and if you can handle the interview then that is the first step along the way!'*

> **Similarly, Samantha (in her second year as a child nurse) had never been to an interview before but recounts:**
>
> *'One comment (that my now personal tutor!) made to me at an open day stuck with me throughout and gave me the belief that I had just as much chance as anyone of being accepted. She asked, 'why shouldn't it be you?' I'll never forget that.'*

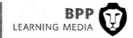

Chapter summary

This chapter has taken a step-by-step approach to selecting a university and making an application. Use the resources identified to guide you in your quest and think through what is going to help you to make a successful application to the university of your choice. The chapter has been complemented by contributions from current students who were where you are not that long ago. They were all keen to encourage you by relating their own experiences in gaining a place. Perhaps the inspiring words that Sam recalled will apply to you too - *'why shouldn't it be you?'*

Key points

- Take time to do your background research and draw up a shortlist of universities that you are interested in. Visit the universities of your choice armed with a list of questions that you want to ask.

- Make sure that you understand both the UCAS application system and what selection process your chosen universities use.

- Take care in writing a personal statement that reflects you as an individual and really focuses on how your life and work experiences relate to your chosen field of nursing. Don't waffle!

- Do not underestimate the importance of thorough preparation for your interview / selection day.

- Remember that getting the right 'fit' is a two-way process – the university wants to select students who will make the most of the opportunities they offer and you will want to choose somewhere where you will be happy and can flourish both personally and professionally.

Useful resources

BBC health web pages: www.bbc.co.uk/health

The Complete University Guide: www.thecompleteuniversityguide.co.uk

Department of Health: www.dh.gov.uk

Nursing and Midwifery Council: www.nmc-uk.org

–   Nb guidance on professional conduct for students can be found at www.nmc-uk.org/Documents/Guidance/Guidance-on-professional-conduct-for-nursing-and-midwifery-students.pdf

Royal College of Nursing: www.rcn.org.uk

UCAS: www.ucas.ac.uk

References

Cameron J, Roxburgh M, Taylor J and Lauder W. Why students leave in the UK: an integrative review of the international research literature. *Journal of Clinical Nursing* 2011; 20(7-8): 1,086-96.

Glogowska M, Young P and Lockyer L. Should I go or should I stay? A study of factors influencing students' decisions on early leaving. *Active Learning in Higher Education* 2007; 8(1): 63-77.

Mclaughlin K, Moutray M and Muldoon O. The role of personality and self-efficacy in the selection and retention of successful nursing students: a longitudinal study. *Journal of Advanced Nursing* 2008; 61(2): 2,011-21.

Nursing and Midwifery Council (2008) *Good practice guidance for selection of candidates to pre-registration nursing and midwifery programmes.* [Online] Available at: www.nmc-uk.org/Documents/Circulars/2008circulars [Accessed 19 January 2012].

O'Donnell H. Expectations and voluntary attrition in nursing students. *Nurse Education on Practice* 2011; 11(1): 54-63.

Taylor R. Creating a connection: tackling student attrition through curriculum development. *Journal of Further and Higher Education* 2005; 29(4): 367-374.

Waters A. The question for universities: how can they win the war on attrition? *Nursing Standard* 2010; 24(24): 12-15.

BPP
LEARNING MEDIA

Chapter 7

Mature or graduate entry nursing

Sue Thompson

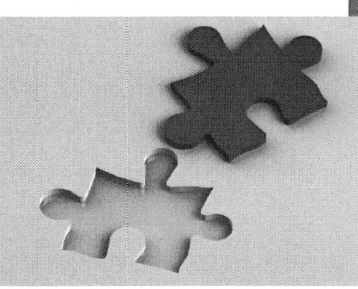

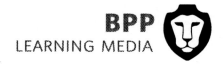

Introduction

Deciding to change direction and take on a new challenge can be a daunting prospect and obviously needs careful consideration. Leaving behind a secure (if not perhaps satisfying), job to take on a demanding programme of education and career is of course a risk. Yet it is a popular one, around one in five new entrants to higher education are classed as mature students, (ie over 21 years of age) and traditionally nurse education takes a high percentage of mature entrants, (Higher Education Academy, 2009). People enter nursing from a wide variety of backgrounds, experiences and age ranges. People may have always harboured the desire to be a nurse from childhood, but got sidetracked, or they may have recently come to the decision, possibly following the illness of a friend or relative. Whatever has brought you to the contemplation of nursing as a profession, the following chapter hopefully will provide you with enough information for you to assess what nurse education and nursing is like for the mature entrant, allowing you to reach an informed decision regarding whether to train and also which course may best suit your needs.

The benefits of being a mature entrant

There are many benefits of being a mature entrant into nurse education, which go a long way to mitigate any sense of 'coming a little late to the party' that mature entrants may feel. Both educators and future employers are well aware of the specific assets that mature entrants tend to bring with them. Chief amongst these is obviously life experience, whether this is through working life or meeting personal challenges. Mature students tend to be more assertive, more focused, have better time management, multi tasking abilities and organisational skills than their younger counterparts. (Kevern and Webb, 2004).They have also been shown to have greater communication skills, essential both for academic work and also interactions within the healthcare environment with patients, carers and colleagues, (Archer, 1999). Research has shown that mature students have greater ability in problem-solving and more self awareness in regard to their strengths and weaknesses than younger students and tend to study at a deeper level, (Saunders and Sadler-Smith, 1996).

Graduate entry nurses having already completed a degree programme come to nurse education with already honed research, debating and critical analysis skills gained during their undergraduate programmes. This together with a knowledge of the structure and expectations of academic programmes help them settle into nurse education quickly (Lizzo and Wilson, 2004).

Mature entrants are also more likely than those in the younger age group to have had practical caring experience – this may be as an healthcare assistant, a volunteer or even a personal carer. Such qualities and experience stand mature students in good stead to achieve a high level of performance academically and in practice, as well as giving mature entrants an insight into the role of the nurse. Obviously if you can, it is better to gain experience in the field of nursing you are choosing to study, but this isn't always possible and any experience either paid or voluntary is beneficial to your application to a greater or lesser extent. As a mature student you are perhaps better placed to gain experience than younger applicants as many healthcare roles are restricted to those above the age of 18 years.

Once qualified, mature graduates or post graduates are more likely to stay within the local geographical area due to family ties and commitments. This represents a good investment on behalf of the training institution. For their part, mature entrants have usually given a lot of time and thought to their decision to become a nurse, and as a result are likely to be highly committed and motivated to succeed and consequently often perform better in both course work and examinations compared to younger students. (McCarey *et al*, 2007)

'The mature students that I have met on the course have all brought different experiences to nursing and I feel that the mix of mature students and students just finishing college is a very healthy thing for nursing and the student nursing experience.' **Sam Humphreys, Student Nurse, University of Nottingham.**

Issues for mature entrants

Mature entrants to nurse education and higher education generally perhaps feel the need to succeed rather more starkly than their younger counterparts, and some students may see nurse education as 'their last chance'. This perhaps is a double edged sword, the pressure encouraging mature students to work hard, but also putting them under greater stress.

Mature students often tend to bond with the other mature students on their course and this can provide an excellent support network. However, mature students can often find themselves falling into a 'mothering role' with the younger students (Steele *et al*, 2005). It may be tempting to adopt this role, however this may not necessarily be in the best interests of the younger students and may distract you from pursuing your own goals.

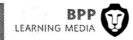

Despite the transferable skills mentioned above that mature entrants bring to higher education, many feel a lack of confidence in the early stages of the course (Kevern and Webb, 2004). A contributing factor to this may be if they have been out of the educational environment for a number of years, and therefore have a lack of familiarity with and / or no prior experience of the higher education sector. Mature entrants to graduate entry nursing courses despite their previous higher educational experience may also suffer from this lack of confidence, possibly due the time elapsed since their degree qualification or if they perceive that the subject taken at undergraduate level fails to prepare them for nursing. Graduate entry nursing courses are accelerated courses, being two years instead of the usual three years, and this may further compound this lack of confidence with the fear the they won't achieve what they need to do within this condensed time frame.

Starting any new enterprise is daunting and the best advice you can follow is to trust the selection process on your course. Universities are penalised if students fail to complete courses, therefore it is in no one's interest to recruit students onto courses about whom there are doubts as to their ability to complete. Nursing lecturers have a duty of care enshrined within their professional nursing registration to ensure that all nurses qualifying from their courses have met the requirements both academically and clinically.

Juggling studying and a nursing career with family and personal life

Financial issues and childcare commitments were shown to be the two areas which caused most concern for mature students, (Montgomery 2009). Until you actually start such a demanding programme of study, you can only guess at the time and financial constraints that will impact on you throughout the course. An essential starting point for mature entry students considering starting or returning to higher education, is to gain the unwavering support of partners and family members. Financial pressures, shift working, needing to find time to study, and travelling to placements, will all take their toll and lead to tiredness and stress. Without a supportive family, who can help with the tasks which possibly had previously fallen to you, it will be extremely hard for you to satisfactorily complete the course. Research shows that women especially can suffer from the expectation that they will continue with their traditional roles, despite the new pressure of studying. Some male partners perceive this new enterprise as more of a hobby for their female partners, as opposed to an investment in the future, (Norton, 1998). Research has shown that a supportive partner is the single most important factor for success for mature students, (Norton, 1998; Steele *et al*, 2005). It is important that this support continues for the duration of the whole course as if support declines, the pressure on mature students to withdraw from the course increases (Norton, 1998).

Shift working

During your course you will be required to work shift patterns (see the *Learning for practice and learning in practice* chapter). This is necessary so you can experience the complete picture of the caring environment and, as we know people don't suddenly get better in the evening, nursing is a 24-hour a day profession. It can be hard to juggle family responsibilities with shift working, but nursing is not necessarily any worse than any other job in this respect. You may for example be able to request certain shifts at certain times, to allow you to see your child's nativity for instance, something that might be more difficult if you had a 9am to 5pm Monday to Friday job. In this, forward planning is the key. Duty rotas are usually prepared at least six weeks in advance and requests need to be made early if they are to have any chance of success. Even then patient care comes first and too many requests for certain times (eg holiday periods) will mean someone at least will be unsuccessful.

Shift working can often work to your advantage. Some practice areas do 12-hour shifts, compressing the working week into less days; night shifts are also often worked one week on, one week off. With most families having two working parents, juggling work and childcare is something common to most families, not just those in the nursing profession.

Holidays

Due to the logistics of running nurse education programmes which encompass both theory and practice time, annual leave for student nurses tends to be set in stone for the duration of the course. When you commence the course, you should be given a plan of the programme which states the annual leave periods. Unlike other university students, generally student nurses don't follow the academic calendar, hence although you will get time off during the summer months, it won't be the long university vacation that students get on other courses, although most schools endeavour to give students Christmas off; Easter, being a movable feast is more tricky.

Obviously once qualified and employed as a nurse, like any other job, you will be allocated a certain number of days per year as annual leave. Annual leave is requested and will be allocated on a rota basis, ie you

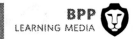

won't be able to have Christmas Day off every year. However, due to the variety of nursing practice, not all practice areas operate a shift system. Community, practice nursing, clinic nursing or working in day centres usually provide more regular hours. It is necessary to bear in mind however, that such areas are popular and jobs in these areas are very competitively sought, precisely because of this factor. Part-time working and job sharing are also widely available within the nursing profession as employers see the need to adopt family friendly employment policies to attract and retain staff.

'I am in my early thirties and have wanted to study nursing for many years, but the trap of well paid jobs always won me over! After having my daughter regular business trips to London, Belfast and Germany lost their appeal. I felt that a more stable career would give me a greater work-life balance. I am approaching the end of my first year (mental health) and have found the transition from full-time work to full-time study really easy to adapt to. This is mainly due to the support and advice available from the university (face-to-face, web-based learning and fellow students). It is a privilege to work alongside health professionals and gain experience interacting with patients, which will equip me with the skills and confidence to practise safely when qualified.' **Sally Wafford, Student Nurse, University of Nottingham.**

Do I have the correct qualifications to start a pre-registration nurse education programme?

Entry requirements

Individual universities will have their own entry requirements which can be found on their websites and in their prospectus. From 2012 all pre-registration nurse education programmes in the UK will be at a minimum degree level. Therefore entry to BSc programmes require level 3 qualifications, that is A levels or equivalent (eg the BTEC National Diploma, the International Baccalaureate etc). In addition nursing courses require entrants to hold GCSE A – C grade English and Mathematics or equivalent, (eg NVQ level 2 numeracy and literacy).

If you are a mature entrant and don't have the required A level equivalent qualifications, another option is to take an Access to Nursing course. These are level 3 (A level equivalent) courses delivered by local further education colleges throughout the UK. Students study a range of health related subjects, for example biology, psychology, sociology, health studies as well as study skills and information technology to prepare them for further study at university level. Courses vary in their entry requirements but you may be required to already have some level 2 (GCSE, BTEC First Diploma equivalent) qualifications. Access courses are free to the under 19's and to those with specific income related circumstances, but otherwise cost around £1,500 with international students paying more. There are a range of courses offered, full- or part-time, one year or two, evening and daytime to fit in with your schedule. If your wish is to proceed from an access course to nurse education make sure the course you apply for is at level 3. Courses do exist at lower levels for students wishing to work in healthcare as support assistants etc, but these will not be at the correct level to gain you access to nurse education.

For those who already have a degree and wish to take a two-year pre-registration post graduate diploma or master's course, individual universities will again set their own entry requirements. Universities may ask for your degree subject to be in a field aligned to nursing – although due to the holistic nature of nursing, this encompasses a broad range of subjects, so don't be put off, it's always useful to enquire regarding your particular course. Courses will also ask you to show evidence of prior healthcare experience in order to demonstrate that you have achieved advanced standing and are therefore eligible for a condensed course. (See FAQs below).

Unsurprisingly given the speed of technical developments in recent years mature entrants can feel out of their depth in technological matters in comparison with younger students. If this is an issue for you, local colleges can provide courses in IT. Key skills essential to acquire before starting a course are producing a document using Word, searching the internet and delivering PowerPoint presentations.

How will I manage financially – what help is available?

Funding

Changes to funding for nurse education courses have recently come into play for courses commencing from 2012 onwards. The good news is that the UK government funds pre-registration nursing courses so there are no tuition fees to pay for any pre-registration course which leads to a registered nursing qualification, whether it be BSc, graduate entry or Master's level. In England, in addition, most students will be eligible for and should receive a small non-means tested bursary, every year. A bursary is a sum of money which you don't have to pay back,

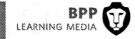

unlike a loan which you do. Also available to those who are eligible is a means tested bursary and a non-means tested maintenance loan. In England these are operated by Student Finance England and for those living in London the amount is increased. The devolved nations have their own funding arrangements. Mature students may be better placed to receive the means tested bursary than younger students still living at home with their parents. It will depend on whether you are living with a partner and what your household income is, as this is taken into account when calculating eligibility. In addition to the basic bursary, students can apply for a number of further allowances if they meet specific criteria. These allowances provide support to disabled students and additional support for students with dependent adults and children. Students can also claim help with travel costs to their placements if they incur additional costs to those incurred when travelling to their university. Further information is available from the NHS Business Services Authority.

Part-time work

Obviously, if you are leaving paid employment in order to take up nurse education, financial considerations will be uppermost in your mind. Nursing courses are very intensive and unlike other degree programmes leave very little room for you to do part- time work alongside them. When you are on practice placement, which you are for 50% of the time, you already work a 37.5-hour week. When in school for the theory component of the course, you will generally find that nursing courses differ substantially from other degree programmes in respect of contact hours / taught content. Whereas a degree in Chemistry or Journalism for example may consist of a maximum of 9 hours a week actually in class, many nursing courses require attendance by students at three or four times that amount of taught theory sessions. The reason for this is that nurse education will provide you with two qualifications, an academic degree and a registrable clinical nursing qualification, which will put you in the position upon qualification of immediately starting work in professional practice.

Nevertheless, student nurses do manage to combine occasional paid work with their studying. Perhaps in this area student nurses have an advantage over non-nursing students as student nurses are considered excellent candidates for healthcare assistant posts, due to their practice experience and educational attainment. Many NHS and private healthcare providers in the UK are able to offer student nurses paid shifts as healthcare assistants on an ad hoc, flexible basis which students can work around their studies and practice placements.

Am I too old?

There is no stipulated upper age limit for commencing nurse education and it is not unheard of to find students beginning nurse education in their 50s. Generally an average cohort of student nurses consists of students aged from 18 years (21 years for graduate entry programmes) to 50 and all ages in between. All student nurses have to have an occupational health screening before commencement on the programme and are screened to ensure they are suitable for admission at that point. The occupational health department also tests students' immune status and keeps them up to date with the required immunisations.

It is important to stress however, that a great deal of nursing practice is physically demanding and requires good energy levels and a degree of physical fitness. Nurses are generally on their feet for much of their shift and walk miles during the course of it. Once you are qualified you may decide to take up a post that is less physically demanding, but during the training programme there is a requirement to rotate around different practice areas. Generally mental health and child nursing are less physical than adult nursing, however as a mental health nurse you may be caring for patients with dementia and children as every parent knows demand a lot of energy expenditure.

Top tip

Get an action plan together before you start, update your skills if you need to, plan when you will do your studying and discuss issues in depth with your partner and family. Find out what financial support you are entitled to and if this will be enough and, if not, explore what part-time working opportunities are available to you. If it is an issue for you, plan childcare arrangements, including emergency arrangements if your child is ill. Many hospitals now have nurseries attached to them and the benefit of using hospital-based facilities is that they cater for nursing shift patterns that some private nurseries or child minders don't. Most schools of nursing are linked to and often on the same campus as regional hospitals in which you may be based for many of your placements, (especially for adult and child fields), so this makes hospital-based childcare facilities very convenient.

Graduate entry nursing

Some universities, for example the Universities of Nottingham and Southampton and King's College London offer a condensed two-year pre-registration nursing programme for those with an existing degree (usually a 2:2 or above).

These courses lead to a post graduate academic qualification – a post graduate diploma and / or a master's degree as well as the standard professional nursing qualification which is registered with the UK Nursing and Midwifery Council (NMC).

Due to the shortened duration, these are intensive full-time courses with a heavy workload and students coming from their first degree, used to minimal contact time and lots of free time to do other things, will experience a shock to the system.

In common with the standard three-year programmes, 50% of time is spent in school and 50% of time is spent in practice. During practice placement time, you will need to complete certain practice outcomes stipulated by the NMC and work a 37.5-hour week. However, like other nursing students you are classed as supernumery – ie not counted within the staffing numbers designated as being necessary for the operation of that ward or practice unit and this leaves you free to pursue your learning needs. Nevertheless, you will obviously be undertaking nursing care and you will be assigned a mentor, a registered nurse who will oversee your practice and assess your achievement of the designated practice outcomes (see the *Learning for practice and learning in practice* chapter).

Case study: An insight into the Graduate Entry Nursing (GEN) course at the University of Nottingham

Graduate Entry Nursing at the University of Nottingham operates out of our Derby centre with placements throughout Derbyshire and North Nottinghamshire. Students apply to study either adult, child or mental health nursing. Students completing the course will gain an MSc in Nursing as well as their registered nurse qualification. This involves the completion of a 15,000-word dissertation for which you will be allocated a supervisor. The programme follows a modular structure. Each module is integrated with clinical placements and is assessed independently, so there are no final examinations. Assignment submission dates are spread throughout the academic year. The modules are designed to complement each other and to build sequentially upon earlier course content. All assignments require students to integrate theoretical and research-based knowledge with critical reflection upon nursing practice. There are seven weeks of holidays each year of the course, with the expectation that students will be actively engaged in study for 45 weeks each year.

The GEN programme seeks to build on the student's prior learning both academically and in practice and as well as having first degree, you will be expected to show experience of working or volunteering in a healthcare environment for a minimum of nine weeks prior to starting the course.

Enquiry-based learning

A key tenet of the GEN programme is self-directed learning, specifically through use of enquiry-based learning. For this you are allocated to a small student group and with a lecturer as a facilitator you are introduced to real-life practice-based scenarios (often in video format). From these you extrapolate your own individual learning needs and research knowledge and issues to share and debate with your group. Enquiry-based learning is complimented by traditional lectures, clinical skills sessions and workshops to endeavour to cater for all learning styles.

Clinical supervision

While you are on placement you are invited back into school every two weeks for a clinical supervision session. These, again in small group format, provide you with an opportunity to discuss practice issues with your peers on the course and lecturers who facilitate the sessions. Nursing is a stressful profession and clinical supervision provides you with a confidential and supportive forum for discussing concerns, as well as an opportunity to explore best practice solutions.

Working alongside medical students

The Shared Family Study is an innovative project in which you are paired up with medical students and assigned to a patient and their family. The patient will have a long-term condition and your role is to assess the psycho-social impact that this condition has on the patient and their family. This involves visiting the patient in their home, talking with them and their relatives and then presenting a poster presentation on one key aspect of their lives.

Why do people undertake a graduate entry nursing course?

'I undertook quite a broad degree which didn't specifically qualify me for a particular occupation. I was fortunate to gain a post working for Social Services as a Day Service Co-ordinator, however, without a professional qualification I wasn't able to gain professional status or increased pay banding. Nursing appealed to me due to the 'hands on' patient contact still associated with the profession in comparison to the paperwork restraints of social work'. **Laura Batterbee, Student Nurse, University of Nottingham.**

A slightly different student experience

'I didn't move into the residences available on campus nor did I share a house with any fellow students as I was already living in the city when I applied to the course. Part of me does feel that I have missed out on the social aspect of the student lifestyle by not moving away from home, however I don't feel that my experience of the course itself has been affected at all.' **Sam Humphreys, Student Nurse, University of Nottingham.**

Graduate entry nursing frequently asked questions

Q: Aren't I better just doing the three-year course?

A: If you have a degree, you are well placed to enter a post graduate (GEN) shortened course. This way you will gain a higher academic qualification and still gain the practice skills necessary for you to qualify. Graduates, due to their life experiences and experience of already being in the academic environment are able to 'hit the ground running' and are well able to gain the necessary skills required for practice without needing the settling-in period perhaps essential for younger, less experienced students.

Q: Can I still live at home and travel to my placements? I don't want to live in halls of residences or in student houses.

A: Well this obviously depends on where you live in relation to your school of nursing and most importantly your practice placements. The amount of travelling required will vary depending on the nature of practice placements utilised by your school, some within a big city may be very local, others based in a rural county will involve a lot of travelling in order for you to gain the required range of placements. Also, mental health care is primarily made up of small community-based services and these may be scattered amongst the various local communities. Child field placements may often include specialist placements which are only available at regional centres, requiring travelling some distance. Being able to drive and have access to a car may prove to be essential, after all many nursing shifts start at 7am and late shifts finish around 9pm. This means that you can drive to work and back out of rush hour periods which is a bonus, but relying on public transport at these times may not be a option. Your university should grant you travelling and parking expenses for travel in excess of the local hospital and nursing school.

Q: Do I need a health related degree?

A: Most graduate entry programmes do not stipulate this as an entry criteria, or may say that it is preferable. It is worth asking individual universities whether your particular degree counts. It is generally acknowledged that having a first degree will give candidates many transferable skills relevant to nursing and you may be asked to demonstrate these transferable skills on application. Nursing is an holistic profession and nurses require many attributes in order to deliver person-centred care, so someone with a Biological Sciences degree or a Psychology degree isn't necessarily looked on any more favourably than a candidate with an English Literature degree for example. It will depend on the skills, qualities and experience that the individual candidate exhibits.

Q: Do I need healthcare experience to get on the course?

A: Most shortened, graduate entry courses require you to demonstrate prior learning relevant to nursing before starting. Due to the shortened nature of the programme and to comply with NMC Assessment of Prior Learning (APEL) requirements, schools will ask you to detail your previous experience. Different university schools vary in the way they ask for this information, so it's best to refer to the entry criteria of the university to which you are applying. As well as this being a requirement, this demonstrates both your commitment and provides you with a level of understanding as to the nature of the role before you take the plunge.

Q: What will the nurses on my practice placement think of me when they find out I've got a degree?

A: This was a common concern for students when graduate programmes started, however more and more registered nurses have degrees themselves now. From 2012 all pre-registration nursing programmes will be degree level at least, so from 2015 all newly qualified nurses will have a degree and those already in practice are increasing their academic qualifications to keep pace. Registered nurses who will support you on placement have a recognised professional qualification, they have experience in the practice area and skills to pass on to students, they therefore welcome students who are enthusiastic and eager to learn and also those who question and challenge.

Q: Am I likely to get a better job or career because I'll get a post graduate qualification?

A: A difficult question to answer, it depends on you. Graduate programmes, as they are at master's level, expect students to work at that level. This means that students are encouraged to question, think critically and analyse. These are excellent leadership skills and lead new registrants to propose and manage new initiatives for their practice areas. Such qualities will get you noticed and may lead to career progression. Of course this is not to say that nurses graduating with diploma or degrees won't also have these skills, so it is largely up to the individual. Practice managers tend to look wider than the academic qualification when they recruit, as they are looking for competent, hard working professionals, but having initiative and spark will be much in your favour.

Away from the practice environment, for those wishing to go into research or teaching a post graduate qualification is an excellent first step.

Chapter summary

Making a career change into nursing is a daunting prospect, but one that hundreds of people make successfully each year. As we have seen existing skills and experience that you may already have acquired, such as assessment, problem-solving, working with people and communication skills are essential and easily transferable to nursing. Although beginning nurse education as a mature entrant is challenging, nursing is an intensely rewarding occupation. Once qualified a range of opportunities open up to you to specialise in areas of particular interest, as well as possibly being able to work in a role that best suits your own particular circumstances.

Key points

- Entering nursing as a mature entrant can be challenging – carefully assess your level of motivation and ability to stay the course.

- Planning is essential for success – you will need to consider whether you will be able to manage financially and how you will juggle work and family commitments.

- On-going emotional and practical support from partners and family is essential.

- Your pre-existing skills and experience will be invaluable – believe in your ability to succeed.

Useful resources

NHS Professionals part-time work
www.nhsprofessionals.nhs.uk

The Nursing Times
www.nursingtimes.net/making-the-most-of-nurse-training/1847884.article

UCAS – Choosing the right course for you
www.ucas.com/students/choosingcourses/specificsubjects/nursing

Scullion, P and Guest, D (2007) *Study Skills for Nursing and Midwifery Students.* Maidenhead: McGraw Hill Education.

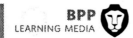

References

Archer, J, Cantwell, R and Bourke, S. Coping at university: an examination of achievement, motivation, self-regulation, confidence, and method of entry. *Higher Education Research and Development* 1999; Volume 18(1): 31-54.

Higher Education Academy (2009) Mature students in higher education and issues for widening participation. HEA evidence net 2009. [Online] Available at: http://evidencenet.pbworks.com/w/page/19383511/Mature%20 students%20in%20higher%20education%20and%20issues%20 for%20widening%20participation [Accessed October 2011].

Kevern, J and Webb, C (2004). Mature women's experiences of pre-registration nurse education. *Journal of Advanced Nursing*, 45(3): 297-306.

Lizzio, A and Wilson, K (2004) First-year students' perceptions of capability. *Studies in Higher Education*, Volume 29(1): 109-128.

McCarey, M, Barr, T and Rattray, J. Predictors of academic performance in a cohort of pre-registration nursing students. *Nurse Education Today* 2007; Volume 27: 357-364.

Montgomery, LEA, Tansey, EA and Roe, SM. The characteristics and experiences of mature nursing students. *Nursing Standard* 2009; 23(20): 35-40.

Norton, B. 'From teaching to learning: theoretical foundations'. In D M Billings & J A Halstead (1998) T*eaching in Nursing: A Guide for Faculty*. 2nd edition. Philadelphia, PA: Elsevier. pp. 211-245.

Saunders, WB and Sadler-Smith, E. Approaches to studying: age, gender and academic performance. *Educational Studies* 1996; Volume 22(3): 367-379.

Steele, R, Lauder, W, Caperchione, C, and Anastasi, J. An exploratory study of the concerns of mature access to nursing students and the coping strategies used to manage these adverse experiences. *Nurse Education Today* 2005; Volume 25: 573-581.

Chapter 8

How do I manage my finances as a student?

Alison Barnard, Zoe Smith, Nicola Siddall, Emma Taylor, and Aimee Aubeeluck

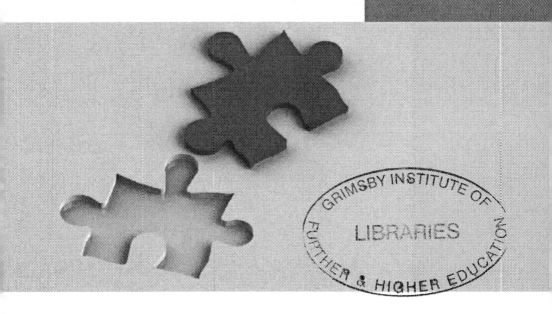

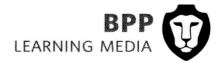

BPP
LEARNING MEDIA

Introduction

This chapter will provide you with an outline of NHS student support and advice on managing your money. If you are new to university or returning to university for graduate entry nurse education, this chapter will offer you some top tips on how to balance the books throughout your course alongside some real-life experiences of managing your money as a student nurse.

Case study: Emma Taylor completed a graduate entry nursing course in 2011:

Unsure of my direction when graduating from university with a degree in Psychology, I worked in a care home for older adults. I soon realised that this was the career that I was destined for; I felt extremely lucky that work did not feel like a chore, and I looked forward to going to work. Soon into my career, I thought about my nurse training, however having a full-time job that I would have to give up, resulting in financial instability, was a significant barrier to me applying to do my training – would it be financially possible to engage in educational endeavours full time?

Having researched what financial help would be available, and discussing this with my manager who offered me flexible part-time hours throughout my training, I applied and gained a place on the graduate entry nursing programme. Receiving a bursary monthly took away the worry of paying rent and utility bills, however this did not leave enough to 'live,' and making such vast lifestyle changes were difficult. I sought advice from the university; and I was supported in applying for and receiving 'access to learning funds', a means tested hardship loan. This money supported me in placement costs and in travel costs to university.

While on practice placement, I soon realised that I was unable to work in my care job, as I did not want to jeopardise my learning opportunities. I settled into the routine of working part-time while studying the theory side of nursing, and full-time in the academic holidays; saving money for the times I would be out on placement. Having a job with hands-on experience eased the financial strain, enabled me to develop personally and professionally, and put my skills and knowledge into practice while out of practice placement. It also enhanced my motivation, as I was working towards my goal.

The academic demands of the course were intense, and it was difficult to balance time in employment and independent study time.

Not having the correct balance could have put my academic achievements at risk; therefore I looked at ways to ease the financial strains of the course. During term time, myself and some fellow students who lived close by began to car share to and from university; which reduced my travel costs by half. Furthermore, while on placement, I claimed back my travel costs on a weekly basis, to ensure that I was not left short. It was difficult; however I made lifestyle changes including where I shopped for my food and how frequently I went out socialising.

It is essential to still engage in the activities you enjoy outside of your nurse training, as the course is not only financially demanding; it is emotionally demanding. Being in the same boat, friends on my course and I ensured we had enough money to socialise at the end of each academic term, to celebrate our achievements, and in between, found 'free activities' to engage in.

There were some incentives, including student discount, NHS discount, reduced council tax and financial help with prescriptions… researching on the internet what financial help is available and the discounts available can ease the financial strain! The motivational incentives of reaching my goal outweighed the financial strains of the course, and although it is difficult, it is possible and it was the best career move I have made.

NHS student support

The review of the NHS bursary scheme, which provides financial support to student nurses has decided that eligible students will all have access to the same package of financial support from September 2012 irrespective of the course that they are taking (Department of Health, 2011). This new package will provide students with a small non-means tested bursary and a reduced rate non-means tested loan. Different rates of means tested bursary and loan will apply according to where a student lives and studies. Some nursing students do manage to have a part-time job that fits around their studies but with a nursing course, it is important to remember that you will be required to work a range of shifts as well as nights and weekends so part-time work needs to be flexible to accommodate the weeks when you are out on placement.

> **Student Nurse Kirsty Fletton found it difficult but possible to make things work financially for her:**
>
> *'I have found the student bursary essential through my first two years; I really don't know how I would have coped without it, even with my Saturday job. Luckily I can say I know when to stop shopping, just, and I have saved a sufficient amount of money through my two years to get me through my final year. The best advice I can give to anyone starting their course is to start saving! You don't want to get to your final year and have no money to buy that amazing graduation dress you have your eye on!'*

'Be prepared'

Just like a good scout, a new student needs to be prepared for the journey they are about to take, and this includes being financially prepared.

Student nurses are no exception to this, so before you start your course it is worth taking the time to make sure you are going to receive all the financial support you are entitled to, and create a budget for the months ahead! Time spent sorting this out now means you will save time (and probably money) over the next few years.

Sounds scary? Well it isn't really. Here are some simple steps to start with:

1. Apply for funding from the NHS Student Bursaries Team

2. You may be able to apply for a student loan from the Student Loans Company – this loan is a fixed amount, is not income assessed and is called the 'reduced rate' loan

3. Make sure you apply for any supplementary grants (Childcare Allowance; Parents Learning Allowance; Dependants Allowance)

4. Do all this **before** you start your course

5. Once you have all the funding award letters in front of you outlining how much you will receive, then you can begin to sort out your budget!

> **Student nurse Sally Wafford agrees,** *'Before accepting my university place, I researched all the available finances from student bursary to child tax credits.'*

Sally makes a good point about child tax credits. If you have children you will still be eligible for this credit, but make sure you tell HMRC that you will be starting a university course. If you have been receiving working tax credit then this is likely to stop. For more information on tax credits go to the Direct gov website(www.direct.gov.uk).

Time to budget

The importance of creating a budget cannot be stressed enough. Research shows that taking control of your money impacts on your physical and mental well being.

> *'There is a strong association between financial capability and psychological wellbeing and also between changes in financial capability and changes in psychological wellbeing. We find that greater financial incapability is associated with greater mental stress, lower reported life satisfaction, and a greater likelihood of reporting health problems associated with anxiety or depression'* (Taylor *et al*, 2009).

How you create your budget isn't important. There is no right or wrong way, the key is to do it. You may find using budgeting tools useful, for example online calculators, or you may prefer to use a simple spreadsheet. There are several 'apps' for smart phones that can be downloaded free of charge. How you do it doesn't matter, just **do it**!

Remember your funding will be paid at irregular times. Any NHS bursary will be paid monthly, whereas student loans are paid termly (three times a year). So you need to get to grips with managing this, particularly if you are used to receiving all your income monthly. You may be giving up paid work to commence your course and it is likely that you will be taking a drop in your income. Careful planning and budgeting will help you deal with the reduction in available cash. Things may be tight financially for a few years, but always keep in mind that once you have graduated you will have a new career ahead of you.

By working out your weekly (or monthly) income and expenditure you can quickly and easily see in black and white whether you have surplus income, or a shortfall. If you have a surplus that's great, but remember to build into your budget an amount for 'miscellaneous', for those unexpected costs that are bound to occur.

If you have a shortfall, **don't panic**! Many students will have a shortfall when setting a budget. If you look at ways to tackle the shortfall before you start your course you will not have to deal with money worries while you are studying. So how can you do this?

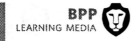

Here are some suggestions:

Top tip

- Find a part time job (you will need some ward experience before you can sign up with NHS Professionals or a nursing 'bank'). Student nurse Sam Humphrey found working a useful way of helping his financial situation. '*Some students (myself included) have a job or pick up work in our free time doing bank shifts as care assistants and support staff. Not only is this a way of increasing your earnings but it's a way a gaining additional experience in one of the most fundamental nursing practices – care.*')

- Cut back on non-essential spending

- Buy basics food items rather than branded

- If you have a student bank account check you have an interest free overdraft available (stay within any agreed limit as going over is likely to incur charges)

- Buy second-hand course books

- Work out how much cash you need per week and only draw that amount out

- Don't take your debit card with you on a night out

Here is what Sally has to say; '*I considered my budget carefully taking into account the local arrangement with the council for reduced or no charges for council tax while studying full time. By setting up direct debits for all my utility bills and shopping around for the best deals, I was able to keep my monthly outgoings down. Check with HMRC to see if you are entitled to a refund of any overpaid income tax. I try to save a little each month, 'rainy day' money' for the unexpected costs that may crop up. Reducing your wants and desires for new and shiny goods also helps you to stay on track with a tight budget!*'

Travelling to placements

Students who receive a means tested bursary from the NHS can apply to be reimbursed with additional 'travel costs'. What does this actually mean? When attending placements your travel costs may be higher than you would normally incur to attend university (where your course lectures and seminars are held). If this is the case then the NHS will reimburse you with any **additional** cost. However you will have to pay the money out first, so remember to include this when planning your budget.

Not all students will be reimbursed though. If your bursary letter shows that your parents / partner are expected to contribute all of your bursary then it is possible they will be expected to cover additional travel costs too.

Debts

If you already owe money to banks or companies (eg store cards or loans) it is important to make sure your repayments are at an amount that you are going to be able to afford while you are studying. If you need help with this, you can seek advice from the Citizens Advice Bureau or similar organisations. The important thing is to sort this out before you start!

Case study: Nicola Siddall, completed a graduate entry nursing course in 2011:

'For me, trying to manage financially was probably the hardest thing about completing the Graduate Entry to Nursing course. I struggled between dedicating enough time to the course alongside a part-time job and having some fun! I obviously received the bursary, without this I would never have been able to complete the course, and this meant I received approximately £550 every third Friday of the month. I also worked as a bank care assistant at a dementia nursing home where I had worked before starting the course. The amount of hours I worked varied greatly, at the beginning I was working up to 30 hours a week but by the end of the course I was only working about 30 hours a month! Having a job related to the course was hugely beneficial. Not only did I earn some money, I was gaining experience in the area that I now work in.

My outgoings generally equalled my incomings and I knew the amount I worked equalled the amount I had to spend on me! I had various people telling me stop drinking on nights out, or to cook instead of getting a takeaway at the weekend, but as far as I was concerned I needed the odd outburst of fun, and personally it was keeping a good social life that kept me sane during the intense periods of the course. Fortunately my boyfriend was extremely supportive and when I moved in with him I didn't have to pay any rent. This helped me hugely. I had various other outgoings which I had to make adjustments to; I adjusted my contract for my phone to the minimum possible, cancelled some not so necessary direct debits, such as internet dongle, gym membership, and a magazine subscription. I also calculated I was spending almost £240 a month on petrol, probably my biggest outgoing, so I made vast changes to the amount I was driving and started walking. This saved on parking too. I made sure I made full use of the NHS travel allowances for all placement driving too.

My other main outgoings were debt repayments. Having previously been an undergraduate before starting nursing I had accumulated debts from two overdrafts, a car on finance, a credit card and a store card. Most of what I was paying back was interest and in hindsight I would have been better consolidating these. The one thing I found hugely beneficial (in some ways) was having a bank account that was not a student account since it made it easier to extend my overdraft for emergencies such as MOTs.

Most importantly, I got sick and tired of people saying "it'll all be worth it in the end" when I was scrimping about for an extra tenner or working seven days a week, but I have to say, they were right!'

And finally

Taking control of your finances now will mean you are less likely to have money worries during your course. If something unexpected does crop up there is always help and advice available at your university. Don't be afraid to contact the relevant department and seek help before you find yourself in a crisis situation. Remember... 'be prepared'.

Case study: Zoe Smith, completed a graduate entry nursing course in 2011:

'When I started my nurse training I had only just finished my three-year degree in Biology at another university, so I was already aware of the challenges of living on a student budget and didn't expect to have any problems. However, during the last two years of my previous degree I had been able to supplement my loan and bursary with a part-time job as a waitress which definitely helped keep me afloat and able to afford the occasional little luxury. It wasn't long after I started placements as a student nurse that I realised it would be very difficult to get another part-time job like that during this degree due to the nature of ever changing shift patterns. Some of my friends worked part-time as agency auxiliary nurses, which suited them very well as it allowed them to work whenever they were able to and also to gain more experience in the field. I remembered though how difficult it had been trying to balance work life, study life and social life before and as I was already doing an accelerated nursing course this time I decided to try and do it without a part-time job.

Having been used to receiving my main income from my student loan and bursary on a termly basis, one thing I found particularly difficult was switching to having my bursary paid on a monthly basis. This was hard as in my first year I lived in student halls where rent was to be paid termly, which fitted in better for all non-nursing students. For the first bursary payment we were given two months in advance, though this was not quite enough to cover the whole first rent payment, and this was where my overdraft came in handy. I know all students like to hope they'll never need to go into their overdraft, but trust me; the overdraft can be your friend if used wisely. Don't be ashamed to use it as long as you don't abuse it (which rhymes, and actually wasn't intentional!). I went to my bank and agreed how much overdraft I was allowed – different banks have different rates for different years of study so that may be worth looking into. I already had a student interest-free overdraft from my previous years of study so I was able to keep it at the same level. For the first few months, I lived in that overdraft until I had been able to save up enough from the monthly bursary payments to scratch my way out of it.

The important thing I found was to try not to worry about it too much. That may sound counter-intuitive and not like what you might have been told, but for me, I find that the more I worry about money and count every penny and try not to spend it, the more likely I am to find myself online buying myself something unnecessary to try to cheer myself up. What I found works best for me was to keep the money issue right at the back of my mind, to know how much I get a month and what definite payments are coming out (rent and phone bills and weekly food allowance) and then roughly how much is left, and just be sensible. I bought basics food ranges from supermarkets, only took a limited amount of money on nights out, didn't splash out on clothes I didn't need without checking my bank balance first, and used the library for books instead of buying them. These habits have stuck with me even though now I'm earning!

A word of warning though, the only time I had to borrow money from my mum (which I still feel guilty about as she refuses to let me pay her back) was at the end of my course. In between finishing the course (and therefore no bursary payments) and starting my new

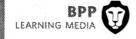

job, I had to wait a few months for all the paperwork and CRB checks to come through, and then one month after starting work to get paid, and I had only budgeted for two months without income before my overdraft limit would start to look a little too close for comfort. You don't know how long you may have to go without income after finishing the course so make sure to factor that time into the budget!'

Chapter summary

This chapter has provided an outline of NHS student support and advice on money management alongside top tips from students. The intensive nature of nursing programmes can leave little time for additional work so balancing your books throughout your course will be key to your success. It can be tough but it **is** possible!

Key points

- Work out how much cash you need per week and only draw that amount out.
- Keep a note pad of all your expenditure and cut back on non-essentials.
- Find a flexible part-time job.

Useful resources

Gov.uk
www.gov.uk/browse/education

NHS Student Bursaries
www.nhsbsa.nhs.uk/816.aspx

Student Loans Company
www.slc.co.uk

References

Department of Health (2011) *Review of NHS Student Support outcome.* [Online] Available at: www.dh.gov.uk. [Accessed 12 April 2012].

Taylor, M, Jenkins, S, and Sacker, A (2009) Financial capability and wellbeing. Evidence from the *British Household Panel Survey*, Financial Services Agency (FSA), UK.

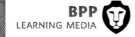
BPP
LEARNING MEDIA

Conclusion

Gemma Stacey, Sue Thompson
and Aimee Aubeeluck

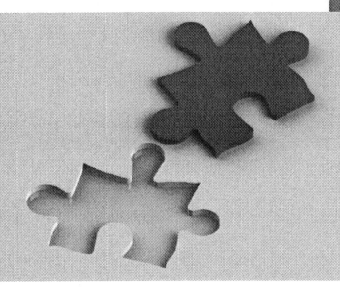

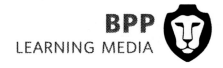

BPP
LEARNING MEDIA

So you want to become a nurse?

You are probably aware that healthcare is a very emotive environment. When people are ill emotions such as fear, grief, anxiety and anger can be very much to the fore, both for patients and their relatives. It is not unusual for nurses to also feel such emotions, nurses after all are expected to care, so it would not be desirable to be emotionless. Nevertheless nurses need to remain in control of themselves and continue to function professionally and effectively, but nursing can be hard sometimes and you need to be able to take care of yourself and build up your resilience. Below is a quote from a student nurse which perfectly illustrates both the joys and distress associated with the role.

'The placements are tremendously varied and can be both challenging and rewarding. One situation that I found hard to come to terms with was when a young woman I was nursing was diagnosed with ovarian cancer, it was devastating news for her family as she had young children. I spent time with the patient and her mum, making them a drink, comforting and supporting them and they were appreciative of this, but that night I went home frustrated and upset, I felt so helpless.

Then again, I remember one particular patient who had suffered a stroke, I spent time reading to him and speaking to his family, and with the involvement of our whole staff team I saw him begin to laugh again, move his head and his hands. I saw him transferred to our local rehabilitation unit. I almost cried with joy because he and his family were doing so well.' **Amy Ward, Student Nurse Adult Field, University Of Nottingham.**

Whatever nursing is, it is neither boring or predictable, but it is challenging and of course tremendously rewarding.

Taking care of yourself through clinical supervision

One way nurses can gain support with the rollercoaster of emotions and events they find themselves part of is via clinical supervision. Clinical supervision is considered best practice amongst registered nurses. It is 'a formal process of professional support and learning which enables individual practitioners to develop knowledge and competence, assume responsibility for their own practice and enhance consumer protection and safety of care in complex situations' (Nursing and Midwifery

Council, 2006). It provides a forum for registered nurses to discuss events and problems, for them to reflect on their practice and systems within practice in order to improve these and make them both safer and more patient-centred. Student nurses while not obliged to undertake clinical supervision can find it beneficial as it provides an opportunity to discuss issues they have encountered in practice, both with their peers on the course and also with a clinical supervisor acting as a facilitator. In this way students are provided with a forum to debate, discuss and work through issues of concern within a supportive environment. Some schools of nursing offer clinical supervision sessions on a regular basis for their students. This provides a valuable opportunity to 'off load', as well as allowing students to question and consider practice they have either observed or been a part of. This includes the sharing of excellent practice as well as poor practice. Having a forum to practise clinical supervision when a student provides an excellent grounding and preparation for clinical supervision once nurses qualify.

Next steps

It is hoped you find this book useful and have now enough information with which to come to the decision 'Is nursing really the career for me?' Hopefully you will now have a clearer idea of the factors you need to consider when choosing nursing as a career. You need to decide which field of nursing would suit you best, which type of pre- registration programme matches your qualifications and experience, which universities to apply to and how to ensure that you gain support in your personal life to enable you to successfully complete a programme of study.

Obviously different readers will be at different stages on the road to commencing a nurse education programme. The table below is designed to take you that one step further, providing you with action points that will fill in the gaps in your knowledge.

	No action needed	Action required	Deadline
I need to obtain additional qualifications			
I need to gain additional experience			
I need to talk to someone for more information			
I need to visit somewhere for more information			
I need to do more research into a specific area			
I need to make changes in my personal life			
I need to look for / talk to people who can support me to do this			

Table 9.1: Action plan

There is no doubt that nursing can be an extremely rewarding career choice. Nurses do truly make a difference to peoples' lives and as such as a nurse you will gain a great deal of job satisfaction. Nursing is often challenging but never boring. Its sheer variety gives you the opportunity throughout your career to care for a wide range of patients with different needs. You also have the option the climb the management ladder, specialise in teaching or research and become a respected advocate for change, influencing policy in your chosen field of expertise.

We all wish you the very best in your nursing career and hope to meet at least some of you in the future.

References

Nursing and Midwifery Council (2006) *Advice Sheet on Clinical Supervision*. London: NMC

BPP
LEARNING MEDIA

Index

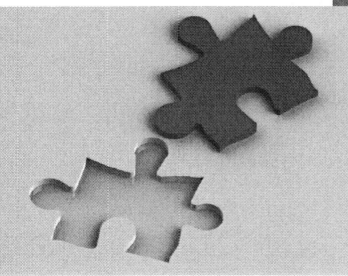

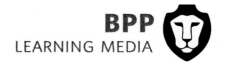

A

B

C

D

E

F

G

H

L